Fundamentals of Clinical Ophthalmology

Cornea

Fundamentals of Clinical Ophthalmology

Cornea

Douglas J Coster

Lions Professor of Ophthalmology,
Flinders University of South Australia,
Flinders Medical Centre, Adelaide, Australia

Series Editor
Susan Lightman
Professor of Clinical Ophthalmology
Institute of Ophthalmology and
Moorfields Eye Hospital, London

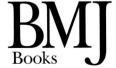

© BMJ Books 2002

BMJ Books is an imprint of the BMJ Publishing Group

First published in 2002
by BMJ Books, BMA House, Tavistock Square,
London WC1H 9JR

www.bmjbooks.com

British Library Cataloguing in Publication Data

A catalogue record for this book is available from the British Library

ISBN 0–7279–1557–6

Typeset by Newgen Imaging Systems (P) Ltd, Chennai
Printed and bound in Malaysia by Times Offset

Contents

Preface to the
Fundamentals of Clinical Ophthalmology series

This book is part of a series of ophthalmic monographs, written for ophthalmologists in training and general ophthalmologists wishing to update their knowledge in specialised areas. The emphasis of each is to combine clinical experience with the current knowledge of the underlying disease processes.

Each monograph provides an up to date, very clinical and practical approach to the subject so that the reader can readily use the information in everyday clinical practice. There are excellent illustrations throughout each text in order to make it easier to relate the subject matter to the patient.

The inspiration for the series came from the growth in communication and training opportunities for ophthalmologists all over the world and a desire to provide clinical books that we can all use. This aim is well reflected in the international panels of contributors who have so generously contributed their time and expertise.

Susan Lightman

Preface

This book is intended to provide a coherent description of disorders of the cornea and their management. Emphasis is placed on diagnosis and, in particular, on the diagnostic process, because accurate diagnosis is essential for effective management.

Although an apparently simple structure, with limited but important functions, the cornea is prone to a wide range of pathological processes. Attention has been directed to the common and important conditions which afflict the cornea. Some less common and perhaps less important conditions are discussed where relevant to the general theme.

This book is intended to be concise. Its aim is to provide an overview, with emphasis on how various conditions relate to one another and on identifying common principles of treatment. For a more detailed discussion of particular conditions there are many monographs and larger textbooks, most of which are disease based and therefore particularly useful after a diagnosis has been made.

Because the cornea is an integral part of the ecosystem of the outer eye, it is unwise to consider it in isolation. The cornea is affected by changes in the conjunctiva, eyelids, tear film and commensal organisms and, conversely, other entities may be affected by changes in the cornea. However, here it has been necessary to consider primarily the cornea and to mention other disorders of the external eye only in passing.

Clinical management implies diagnosis and treatment. Treatment is discussed in general terms in the body of the text and the specifics of treating particular conditions are set out in tabular form in Chapter 15.

Solitary authorship facilitates coherence but increases the threat of personal bias. I have tried to minimise this by basing my views on the evidence provided in the published literature. As with all clinical medicine, however, there are large gaps in the justification of common clinical practices. In such cases, I have had no choice but to present a more personal view but in doing so, I have attempted to present the collective view of experienced clinicians in the field.

Douglas Coster

To BRJ, DBJ and KAW

Acknowledgements

Many people have contributed to this book, some indirectly by teaching and encouraging me and others directly by participating in its production.

I have been privileged through the years to have a number of cherished teachers and mentors, all of whom have been extremely generous with their knowledge and time. I hope they see this book as an extension of their own work. In particular, I wish to acknowledge my debt to Barrie Jones, Dan Jones, Noel Rice, Peter Wright, and Dick Galbraith.

Over the past 20 years, I have been fortunate to have outstanding colleagues at the Flinders University of South Australia who have continued my education. Keryn Williams, Paul Badenoch, and Richard Mills have helped me a great deal, as have the many Fellows and researchers who have spent time with us.

Direct contributions have come from Angela Chappell who took most of the photographs, Nick Hawkesworth who drew the illustrations of corneal transplantation, Wendy Laffer who provided editorial assistance, and Joyce Moore who produced the manuscript.

1 Foundations of keratology

The cornea is an apparently simple structure which can be afflicted by almost the full range of pathological processes responsible for human disease.

Because it requires an undisturbed ultrastructure to function normally in the optical sense, minor disturbances of the cornea can have devastating consequences for vision. Worldwide, corneal disease is second only to cataract as a cause of blindness.

The clear, inert, glass-like appearance of the cornea is misleading. It is a vital tissue with demanding metabolic and cellular requirements for optimal function. Furthermore, it is part of the complex ecosystem of the external eye, which in turn is influenced by general environmental conditions and the body as a whole. Not surprisingly, then, the cornea can be affected by many intrinsic and extrinsic influences.

Much of what is seen as clinical corneal disease is the end result of compromise between the optical and protective functions of the cornea. As a preliminary to considering clinical disease, it is useful to consider the cornea in the broader context of the ocular surface ecosystem which, in turn, is influenced by the general state of the patient and the environment in which the patient lives.

When considering corneal disease, therefore, two notions should be kept in mind because they are central to the understanding of corneal disorders. First, the cornea cannot be considered in isolation but must be thought of as part of the ecological system of the ocular surface. Second, the cornea has two distinct and conflicting functions: an optical function and a protective function. Inevitably, there is compromise and this contributes to the pathogenesis of many corneal disorders. Each of these notions deserves preliminary discussion.

Ecology of the ocular surface

Although it is tempting to think of the cornea as an isolated entity, it is structurally and functionally dependent on associated structures. For this reason, the cornea must be considered in the context of the ecosystem of the outer eye, comprising the cornea, conjunctiva, tear film, eyelids, and commensal organisms of the conjunctival sac (Figure 1.1). Any significant disturbance in one element of the system inevitably affects other elements. For example, infection of the meibomian glands in the eyelids alters the oils secreted into the tear film. This alters the surface tension of the tears and the integrity of the tear film, which in turn influences corneal epithelial nutrition and respiration with subsequent dystrophic changes to the corneal surface. Similarly, damage to the corneal endothelium results in excessive accumulation of water in the cornea and epithelial blisters or bullae. When the blisters unroof, the subsequent corneal ulceration enables the commensal organisms of the conjunctival sac and lid margin to invade the cornea and create an infective focus.

The ecosystem of the ocular surface does not exist in isolation but is influenced by external

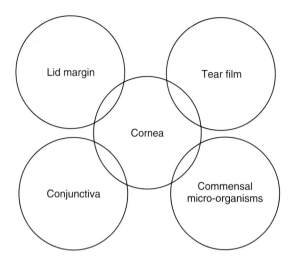

Figure 1.1   Ocular elements comprising the ocular surface ecosystem

factors, both systemic and extracorporeal (Figure 1.2). For example, systemic mucosal scarring disorders such as Stevens–Johnson syndrome and pemphigoid affect the conjunctiva and the tear film. Extracorporeal factors influencing the ocular surface ecosystem include the commensal organisms of the conjunctival sac which vary according to the geographic region. There are more fungal organisms in the conjunctival sac in the humid, tropical regions of the world than are found in temperate climatic

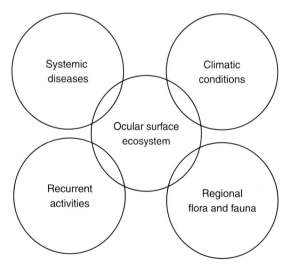

Figure 1.2   External influences on the ocular surface ecosystem

zones. Similarly, different patterns of bacteria responsible for corneal infections in different populations around the world reflect the regional differences in commensal organisms.

There are other ways in which climatic differences can affect the ecosystem of the outer eye. For example, in regions of high sunlight, extreme temperatures, and low humidity, changes induced in the surface of the cornea include climatic droplet keratopathy, pterygium, and pinguecula. Similarly, a person's recurrent activities can affect the ocular surface ecosystem. For example, outdoor rural workers will experience different patterns of ocular surface changes to those experienced by indoor office workers.

Optical role of the cornea

The cornea is an important element in the optical system of the eye, contributing 75% of the refracting power (Figure 1.3). It is crucial to the generation of a high quality image on the retina. For refraction to be accurate and transparency to be maintained, the highly regular ultrastructure of the eye must remain pristine. Even small amounts of oedema, scarring, or metabolic deposits can profoundly affect the optical function of the cornea.

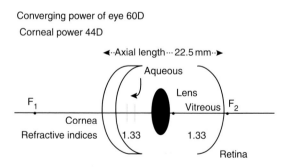

Figure 1.3   The cornea in the optical system of the eye

Protective role of the cornea

The cornea has important protective functions. It protects the internal milieu of the eye from the external environment and is equipped

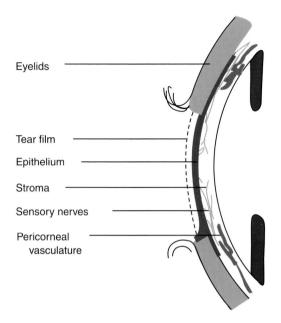

Eyelids

Tear film

Epithelium

Stroma

Sensory nerves

Pericorneal
vasculature

Figure 1.4 Contributions to the protection of the cornea come from the eyelids, tear film, corneal epithelium, corneal stroma, corneal nerves, and pericorneal vasculature

accordingly. The corneal stroma is a thick, tough layer of collagen and, although avascular itself, the cornea is surrounded by a mucosa capable of mounting a brisk inflammatory reaction on behalf of the cornea it abuts. The cornea is richly innervated with sensory nerves and covered by epithelium with extraordinary regenerative capability. All of these protective strategies are, however, potentially damaging to vision. When the cornea is challenged, the protective responses generated can affect the optical properties of the cornea (Figure 1.4).

Conflicting functions, compromise, and corneal disease

It is the compromise between the optical and protective functions of the cornea that is central to many corneal disorders. For example, corneal ulceration and infection generate a brisk inflammatory response which is painful and destroys the normal structural integrity of the transparent cornea, resulting in visual loss. What is seen clinically is the summation of the direct damage caused by the threatening agent, the host response to challenge, and the underlying normal corneal structure.

Because the normal cornea is transparent, abnormalities within it can be seen directly. This was put to good use by Conheim in 1857. His observations of the dynamic nature of inflammation which he induced in the corneas of frogs initiated the current concepts of the inflammatory process. Furthermore, the cornea is conveniently placed for observation with a biomicroscope. Using modern slit lamp biomicroscopes, pathological processes in the cornea can be observed in detail. Virtually all processes occurring in the cornea can be directly observed and many can be observed at a cellular level. For example, the pathological changes in the morphology of the endothelium, recruitment of inflammatory cells from limbal vessels, and the movement of blood cells through capillaries are all readily observed in the clinic.

Ophthalmologists are therefore in a position to observe the interaction of a challenging agent such as infection or trauma and the host response to the challenge, such as inflammation, dysplasia, or neoplasia, and to observe the effect of this interaction on the corneal structure. It is the interpretation of these changes, the way they produce symptoms, and the signs in the cornea and ocular surface which lies at the heart of managing patients with corneal disease.

Diagnosis of corneal disorders

In the clinical context, management implies diagnosis and treatment. Advances in medical therapy have largely been advances in specificity. Effective treatments impact maximally on the disease process and minimally on the normal aspects of the patient's biology. However, specific therapy demands a specific diagnosis. Making an accurate diagnosis is central to all clinical medicine. To achieve an accurate diagnosis demands appropriate thought processes, clinical skills, and knowledge of the biological basis of medicine.

The diagnostic process

Since making an accurate diagnosis is an essential part of clinical practice, it is useful to examine how effective clinicians go about the process. Identifying the key steps in their thought processes will reveal what we need to know to be accurate diagnosticians.

The diagnostic process involves at least four steps (Figure 1.5):

elucidation of clinical features

recognition of major patterns of disease

generation and testing of hypotheses

Elucidation of clinical features: the clinical encounter

Taking a history and examining the patient are fundamental steps in the process of accurate diagnosis. Since most pathology affecting the eye, and particularly the cornea, can be directly observed, it is sometimes tempting for ophthalmologists to pay little attention to the history and to depend on the examination to make a diagnosis. This is a mistake. As with internal medicine, most diagnoses can be made from the history and the examination used more as a confirmatory test. Taking a careful history reveals not only the symptoms of the disease but aspects of the person which are invaluable in planning the most appropriate management for the individual. An appropriate test of the history taking process is for clinicians to ask themselves whether they have made a provisional diagnosis, based on the history, before examining the patient.

The examination of the patient must be complete, with special emphasis on confirming or eliminating suspicions arising from the history. It is important to specifically and deliberately observe the patient as a whole, the face and particularly the periorbital region, before moving to the slit lamp. Common errors are made by moving on too promptly with the

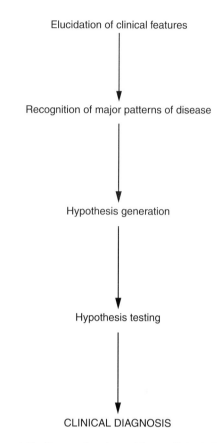

Elucidation of clinical features

Recognition of major patterns of disease

Hypothesis generation

Hypothesis testing

CLINICAL DIAGNOSIS

Figure 1.5   Steps taken in making a clinical diagnosis

examination: for example, not evaluating the ocular surface before instilling mydriatics, not evaluating pupil responses in patients with impaired vision and corneal disorders, or applanating the cornea before testing corneal sensation.

After completing the history and examination comes the process of finding meaning and a diagnosis.

As part of the clinical appraisal, clinicians generate hypotheses which are tested by going back to the patient for more information; asking more questions, looking specifically for clinical signs, and, at the end of the clinical examination, requesting special investigations. The manner of hypothesis generation deserves attention.

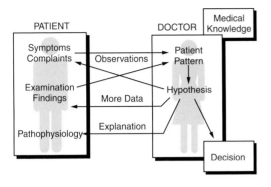

Figure 1.6 Hypothesis generation and making a clinical diagnosis. As information is elucidated in the history and examination, hypotheses are generated and these are continually tested by tracking back to the patient for additional information

Effective diagnosticians are adept at generating and testing hypotheses (Figure 1.6).

Generating and testing diagnostic hypotheses

Hypothesis generation and testing are dependent on the knowledge of the clinician. There are two major components of relevant knowledge. First, clinical experience, where specific information is "arranged" in appropriate patterns reflecting clinical experience. This knowledge is acquired either directly by clinical practice or indirectly from sources such as papers, books, and lectures. Second, knowledge and understanding of biology, which allows the interpretation of clinical findings. It has been estimated that most clinical disciplines require about 2 million "bits" of information for day to day decision making.

Pattern recognition and clinical diagnosis

Experience is an asset in the development of diagnostic acumen. The essential benefit of experience is in the acquisition of new knowledge and the arrangement of existing knowledge so as to assist pattern recognition. This facilitates the comparison of clinical features recognised by the clinician with commonly recurring patterns of clinical disease. Pattern recognition is an important psychological process in many fields of human endeavour and has been extensively studied. It is generally agreed that it depends on parallel processing of information, that we can consider 4–6 elements parallel to one another, and that "hands-on experience" is the most effective way of generating templates with which to compare new observations.

"Hands-on experience" (perhaps "eyes-on experience" is a better term in this context) accrues with time and most clinicians become better clinicians with the passing of the years. However, this is a slow process. Anything which can be learned from experience can be taught by an experienced and generous teacher. Invariably, two qualities which characterise an outstanding teacher are generosity and the willingness to pass on in a few minutes what has been learned over decades, plus the ability to distil the essential from vast amounts of experience.

Pattern recognition involves parallel processing of 4–6 streams of information. Spoken and written description is, by necessity, sequential, so that it is impossible to describe precisely how a clinician goes about the pattern recognition which is at the heart of clinical diagnosis. However, a convenient way of doing this is with diagnostic algorithms. The major advantage of teaching algorithms to inexperienced clinicians is that they provide a framework upon which to lay out experience as it is acquired, accelerating the impact of experience on the development of diagnostic acumen. Various algorithms will be discussed when considering specific clinical entities.

An understanding of the biological principles of disease is also important in providing an explanation of clinical findings. This practical knowledge provides the links between findings and causation and is essential for hypothesis generation and testing. For example, in the context of corneal and ocular surface disease, an understanding of the structure and function of a conjunctival follicle facilitates the generation of diagnostic hypotheses in patients with superficial keratopathy and follicular conjunctivitis. Not only is it important to recognise the difference between a follicle and a papilla in the conjunctiva, but one must also understand the pathobiological significance. A knowledge of pathobiology is also important at a later stage of hypothesis testing when ordering special investigations. For example, a knowledge of likely pathogens is necessary to arrange the appropriate microbiological investigation of a patient with corneal infection.

Knowledge required for diagnostic acumen

In summary, an acceptance of the idealised model of the diagnostic process described above indicates the domains in which clinicians must develop their ability:

Identification of clinical features

Pattern recognition

Hypothesis generation and testing dependent on a matrix of experience and a knowledge of pathobiology

Clinical features of corneal disease

Recognition of clinical features is the first step in managing corneal disease. Without an accurate assessment of the clinical features, the subsequent steps in diagnosis and treatment cannot be taken. Clinical features comprise symptoms and signs.

Symptoms of corneal disease

Pain

Pain is a common feature of corneal disease. It may be due to direct stimulation of the rich plexus of sensory nerves contained in the cornea or the consequence of inflammation or ciliary spasm.

Direct stimulation of the corneal nerves, as occurs in corneal abrasions, results in pain which is severe in intensity and sharp in nature. Inflammation of the cornea, as occurs with corneal infection, can also produce severe pain but of a dull, aching, or throbbing nature.

Corneal disease can also cause photophobia which results in spasmodic pain on exposure to light. This is a consequence of ciliary spasm, particularly if there is associated intraocular inflammation with involvement of the iris.

Chronic corneal diseases, such as herpetic keratitis or chronic epithelial defects, may not be particularly painful or may even be painless, due to denervation in the affected area of the cornea.

Visual loss

Visual loss is common in patients with corneal disease and may be attributable to a number of distinct mechanisms. Loss of transparency of the cornea and alteration in corneal surface shape are also associated with visual loss.

Acute loss of vision is generally due to acute inflammatory conditions of the cornea and is usually associated with other symptoms of inflammation, pain, and vascular injection.

Gradual loss of vision is more likely to be associated with a slowly evolving corneal pathology, such as a change in shape producing a refractive change, as in keratoconus, or the slow accumulation of opacities in the cornea as a consequence of a dystrophy, which is likely to be bilateral, or chronic inflammation, which is more likely to affect one eye.

Visual loss may only be troublesome under certain circumstances. For example, clouding of vision on waking, which reduces through the day, suggests corneal oedema due to endothelial dysfunction. Loss of vision under glare conditions suggests light scatter from relative opacities in the cornea.

Clinical signs of corneal disease

Visual loss

Visual loss as a sign of corneal disease is usually sufficient to register as a reduction in Snellen acuity. Corneal disease can also cause a reduction in contrast sensitivity. Patients may notice a change in visual performance that will only manifest as a reduction in contrast sensitivity under glare conditions. This occurs because forward scatter of media opacities provides a veiling luminance that impairs edge detection and contrast sensitivity.

Slit lamp examination of the cornea

Slit lamp examination is an essential technique for examining the cornea. The cornea is, like all other transparent structures, not entirely transparent. Even the normal cornea has within it structures which refract and scatter the light. Pathological processes tend to produce irregularities which are even more obvious.

The slit lamp, in its essential form, consists of an illuminating beam and a microscope. Each is movable relative to the object to be viewed and to each other. In examining the cornea, the path of the light beam through the cornea is observed. Several distinct but related strategies can be used to enhance the view of the corneal structures. The path of the light beam may be viewed directly as it passes through the cornea or indirectly after it has been reflected off other ocular structures.

Direct illumination with a narrow beam is appropriate for viewing many corneal structures which scatter light. Direct illumination with a broader beam creates specular reflection off irregular membranous structures and is therefore useful for viewing structures such as Descemet's membrane and the endothelium (Figure 1.7).

Indirect illumination of corneal structures can be achieved by illuminating the cornea at the limbus and observing the way light, trapped in the cornea by internal reflection, is interfered with. This technique is referred to as *sclerotic scatter* (Figure 1.8).

Another approach to indirect illumination is to view structures in the beam of light reflected back off the retina (Figure 1.9). A dilated pupil facilitates this approach.

The illuminating beam can also be reflected off relative opacities in the almost transparent cornea. This technique of specular reflection is used to examine the corneal endothelium (Figure 1.10).

In addition to techniques used for visualising the cornea, the slit lamp is used, with the addition

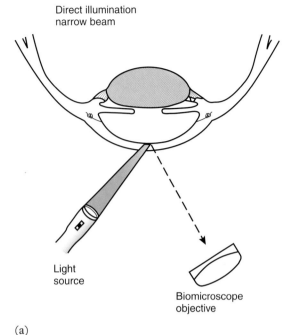

Direct illumination narrow beam

Light source

Biomicroscope objective

(a)

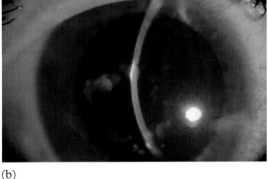

(b)

Figure 1.7(a, b)   Slit lamp examination of the cornea – direct illumination. An optical section of the cornea is illuminated with a narrow or broad slit. A broad slit is used to reflect light off irregular membranes – specular reflection

of the appropriate optical devices, to measure intraocular pressure by applanation, measure corneal thickness with optical pachymetry, and view the anterior chamber and retina with diagnostic contact lenses.

Gullstrand is acknowledged as the originator of the slit lamp, although it may be more accurate to say that he designed an instrument at

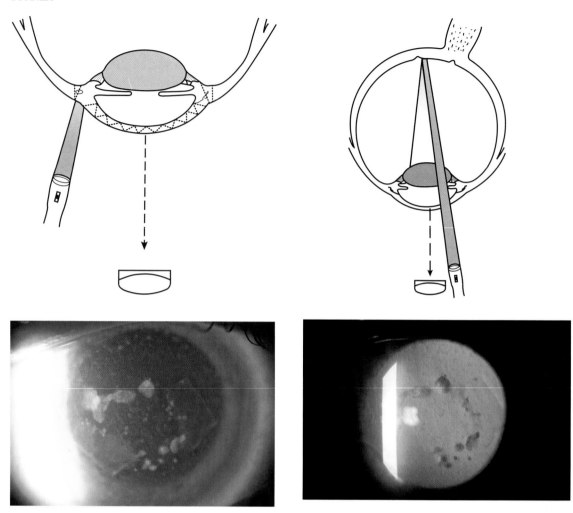

Figure 1.8(a, b)   Slit lamp examination of the cornea – indirect illumination. The cornea is illuminated at the limbus. Most of the light is contained within the area by internal reflection. This technique of sclerotic scatter illuminates opacities in the stroma

Figure 1.9(a, b)   Indirect illumination. Retro-illumination of the cornea is achieved by reflecting light off the retina. A dilated pupil is usually necessary to achieve a satisfactory image

a critical time in its evolution. The evolution of the instrument continues today and current models used by ophthalmologists are very sophisticated.

Corneal ulceration

Loss of the corneal epithelium is a common and sight threatening problem. The extent of a corneal epithelial defect can be seen with the slit lamp and is facilitated by the use of dyes. Fluorescein stains the base of the ulcer and is easily seen, particularly with a blue light. Rose bengal reveals as much and more than fluorescein. It stains the epithelial edge brilliantly without seeping into the stroma and anterior chamber to produce a flare, such as is seen with fluorescein. Of interest to the clinician is the size (which should be measured and recorded in the notes), shape, characteristics of the edge, and the state of the underlying stroma.

In severe cases, not only is the epithelium deficient, with underlying stromal inflammation present, but there may also be loss of stromal tissue. In this situation, stromal lysis is a consequence of stromal inflammation. Descemet's membrane may be more resistant to lysis than the stroma, so that when all of the stroma is lost, Descemet's membrane may persist, creating a descemetocoele.

One situation where corneal lysis occurs without inflammation is in patients with rheumatoid arthritis who develop mid-peripheral corneal ulceration without evidence of inflammation.

Superficial keratopathy

Disturbance of the superficial cornea, that is, the epithelium and its underlying support, occurs in recurring patterns. These include punctate, dendritic, linear, and vortex keratopathy and will be discussed in detail in Chapter 4.

Corneal oedema

Water may accumulate in the cornea, causing an increase in corneal thickness, loss of corneal transparency, and blisters (bullae) in the epithelium. Slit lamp examination will reveal the stroma to be thickened (this can be quantified with ultrasound or optical pachymetry) with a loss of transparency. Epithelial oedema may be seen either as diffuse opacification of a slightly opacified epithelial layer without focal pathology or as bullae (Figure 1.11). In its very mildest form, epithelial oedema produces a diffuse image of the slit lamp beam beside the entrance beam because the oedematous epithelium causes internal reflection of the emerging slit beam within the stroma.

Stromal oedema produces a diffuse opacity, best seen with retro-illumination. The slit beam reflected back off the iris has very soft diffuse edges.

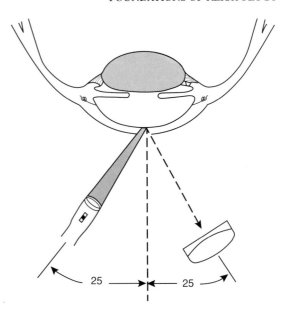

Figure 1.10 Indirect illumination – specular reflection with a broad illuminating beam and the observing and illuminating angle equal, specular reflection of light from membranous structures such as Descemet's membrane and the endothelium is accentuated

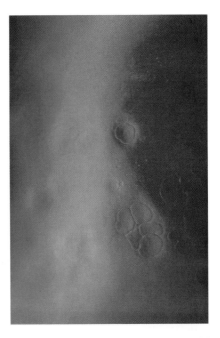

Figure 1.11 Corneal oedema. Blebs filled with cystic fluid (bullae) occur in the epithelium and the slit lamp beam is diffuse in the stroma rather than retaining its normal sharp edges

Acute inflammation of the cornea

The classic changes of inflammation can be seen in the cornea at both a macroscopic and microscopic level. Invariable features are pain, decreased vision, swelling of the cornea due to oedema, opacity due to cellular infiltration, and dilation of vessels in the eye wall and the iris. Slit lamp examination reveals this at a microscopic level. If there is significant involvement of the iris, proteins and cells will enter the aqueous and be seen as flare in the slit lamp beam and circulating cells (Figure 1.12). One consequence of acute inflammation is chronic inflammation.

Chronic inflammation of the cornea

Slit lamp examination will reveal the sequelae of inflammation, with areas of cellular infiltrate, oedema, scarring, and neovascularisation (Figure 1.13). There may also be loss of sensation. In long-standing chronic inflammation, amyloid may deposit in fibrotic areas, creating lumps which may elevate the overlying epithelium. This is called *Salzmann's nodular dystrophy*.

Scarring

Stromal scars appear as opacities within the cornea. They are visible because of back scatter of light and disturb vision because they also cause forward scatter of light. Unlike oedema, scars are seen with sharp edges in the retro-illumination beam (Figure 1.14).

Scarring may also affect the shape of the cornea. Scar tissue contracts with time and this contraction may result in an area of depression or facet in the corneal surface. Irregularities in the anterior refracting surface of the cornea cause degradation of the retinal image and impair vision. The impact of surface irregularities on visual function can be negated by the use of a hard contact lens; this is often a useful clinical trial.

Neovascularisation

The normal cornea is avascular but vessels may develop as a consequence of chronic inflammation or hypoxia (Figure 1.15). Once

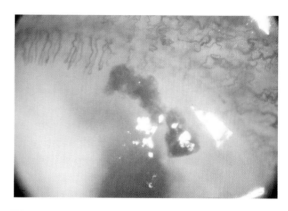

Figure 1.12 Acute inflammation of the cornea. There is oedema, cellular infiltration, dilated limbal vessels, loss of proteins into the cornea and aqueous humour (flare) and egress of inflammatory cells in the anterior chamber

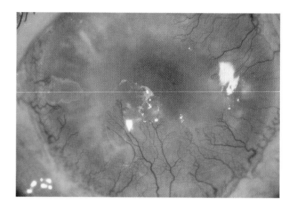

Figure 1.13 Chronic inflammation of the cornea with cellular infiltration, oedema, scarring, and neovascularisation

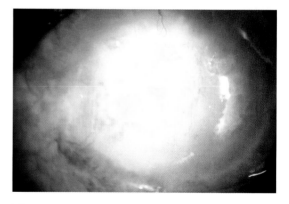

Figure 1.14 Chronic inflammation of the cornea with chronic oedema, cellular infiltration, scarring with calcification, and neovascularisation

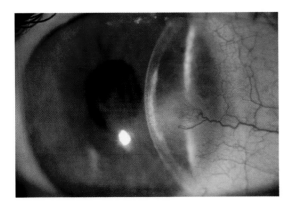

Figure 1.15 Vascularisation of the cornea – a consequence of chronic inflammation or hypoxia

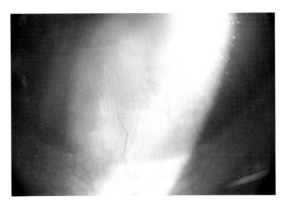

Figure 1.16 Active corneal vessels. The cornea around the vessels is oedematous so that the slit lamp beam cannot be seen in sharp focus. The perivascular oedema is best seen with retro-illumination

the cornea is vascularised, it tends to remain so. With time the vessels may not carry blood but their walls persist. Such ghost vessels, although they may be so attenuated that it is difficult to see them with the slit lamp, will carry blood again should inflammation recur.

New or active vessels may be distinguished from established inactive vessels by their slit lamp appearance. Active vessels are surrounded by an area of stromal oedema. Examining the cornea with retro-illumination reveals a soft-edged mild opacity surrounding the vessels (Figure 1.16). Old inactive vessels, on the other hand, even when carrying blood (that is, not ghost vessels) can be seen to have hard edges when examined with retro-illumination with the slit lamp.

Lipid deposition

Corneal vascularisation can be complicated by lipid extravasation. White or yellow material accumulates in the corneal stroma, usually with a disciform distribution and an obvious feeding vessel (Figure 1.17).

Conjunctival reactions

Many significant corneal disorders are associated with conjunctival changes. Inflammation of the cornea is always associated with some conjunctival injection. In many situations the conjunctival changes accompanying corneal disease may be quite specific. For

example, acute or chronic keratitis may be associated with conjunctival injection and follicles or papillae and chronic corneal disorders may be associated with infiltrative conjunctival changes or submucosal fibrosis. Some of these associated conjunctival changes deserve specific description.

Follicular conjunctival response Follicles are small rounded structures which tend to occur in the conjunctival fornices but which may also occur on the tarsal plate and, rarely, in the bulbar conjunctiva. They can be seen with the naked eye but when viewed with the slit lamp they are a little pale at the apex where the

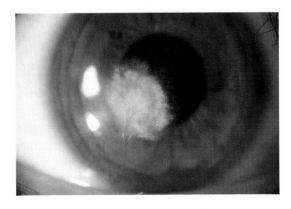

Figure 1.17 Lipid keratopathy with feeding vessels

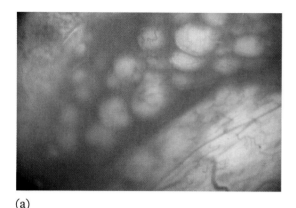

(a)

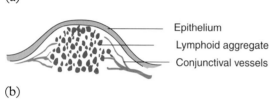

Epithelium
Lymphoid aggregate
Conjunctival vessels

(b)

Figure 1.18 (a) Follicular conjunctivitis. Follicles are aggregates of lymphoid tissue under the conjunctival epithelium. (b) The conjunctival epithelium is stretched, and sometimes blanched, over the aggregation of lymphocyte and other mononuclear cells

conjunctival vessels are blanched by the pressure of the small space occupied. Follicles are aggregations of lymphoid tissue in the lamina propria of the conjunctiva and are a response to chronic drug toxicity or infection with viruses or chlamydia (Figure 1.18).

Papillary conjunctival response Papillae are proliferations of conjunctiva. In their mature form, they are seen as small flat protrusions of conjunctiva containing a central blood vessel with side branches, much like a Christmas tree. The presence of the blood vessel in the central area (where, conversely, the protruding follicle is blanched) and the tabloid shape are characteristic of papillae and distinguish the lesions from follicles. Papillae occur on the tarsal plate and may vary in size. When small, they give the conjunctiva a velvety appearance (Figure 1.19). When large, they appear more like cobblestones. Those more than 2 mm across are described as giant papillae. A papillary response is usually associated with allergic disease or contact lens use (Figure 1.20).

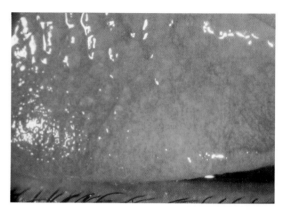

Figure 1.19 Small papillae giving the cornea a velvety appearance

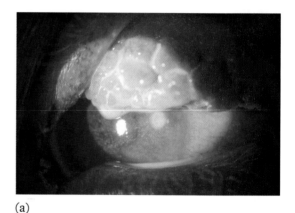

(a)

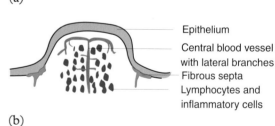

Epithelium
Central blood vessel with lateral branches
Fibrous septa
Lymphocytes and inflammatory cells

(b)

Figure 1.20 (a) Large conjunctival papillae associated with chronic allergic conjunctivitis or contact lens use. (b) Architecture of conjunctival papillae. Papillae are formed around central blood vessels which provide a framework for oedema, acute and chronic inflammatory cells, separated by fibrous septae

Infiltrative conjunctival reaction The conjunctiva can become infiltrated with large numbers of cells, turning the normally thin, mobile membrane into a thicker, stiffer structure. Infiltrative conjunctival changes are found in malignant conditions, particularly haematological disorders such as lymphoma. Infiltrative changes can also be the result of chronic injury such as chemical burns or with chronic inflammation (Figure 1.21).

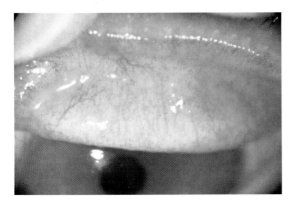

Figure 1.21 Infiltrative conjunctival reaction. The conjunctiva at the ends of the tarsal plate is diffusely thickened. Biopsy revealed lymphoma

Conjunctival subepithelial fibrosis Chronic inflammation of the conjunctiva can result in submucosal fibrosis, seen clinically through the transparent conjunctival epithelium as white scar tissue with fine, fibrillary morphology. Although most obvious when the upper tarsal conjunctiva is involved, it can be seen anywhere. At its most obvious, it appears as a horizontal scar running along the tarsal plate, a clinical feature known for many years as an *Arlts line* and originally described as a feature of trachoma. In severe forms, submucosal fibrosis alters the architecture of the conjunctival sac, the medial canthus usually being affected initially. When severe, it can obliterate the fornices and cause cicatricial entropion.

All causes of chronic conjunctivitis can lead to subepithelial fibrosis but it is most obvious with ocular cicatricial pemphigoid, Stevens–Johnson syndrome and trachoma (Figure 1.22).

Lid conditions associated with corneal disease

The eyelids are important to the cornea. They protect it and are responsible for maintaining and moving the tear film across the corneal

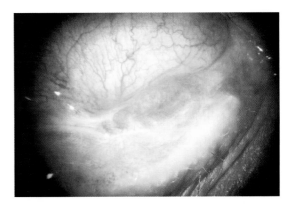

Figure 1.22 Submucosal fibrosis. Linear white scars are seen under the conjunctival epithelium and there is disturbance of the normal surface architecture

epithelium and therefore the nutrition and oxygenation of the superficial cornea. In addition, glandular structures in the lids secrete oils onto the tear film, limiting its evaporation. Not surprisingly, abnormalities of eyelid structure and function are often associated with corneal disease.

Anterior blepharitis Anterior blepharitis results in injection of the vessels of the anterior lid margin, desquamation of the epidermis, which may collect around the base of the lashes as collarettes, and disturbance of lash growth. The lashes may be decreased or absent (*polyosis*) or grow irregularly and in abnormal directions (*dystikiasis*) (Figure 1.23).

Posterior blepharitis Posterior blepharitis involves inflammation of the meibomian glands, altering the nature of the oil they secrete and thereby adversely affecting the tear film and the corneal epithelium. It is a chronic relapsing condition which results in swelling and rounding of the posterior lid margin, dilation of vessels in the same region, plugging of the meibomian gland openings with solidified oils, and scarring as evidence of previous glandular inflammation. Some patients develop features of both anterior and posterior lid margin inflammation (Figure 1.24). Features of anterior and posterior blepharitis are summarized in Table 1.1.

Table 1.1   Features of anterior and posterior blepharitis

	Anterior	Posterior
Microbial elements	Sometimes (staphylococcal)	Rarely
Dystichiasis	Often	Rarely
Polyosis	Sometimes	Rarely
Collarettes	Common	Rarely
Meibomian gland changes	Rare	Common
Lid ulceration	Sometimes	No
Conjunctivitis	Mild	Mild
Keratitis	Punctate epithelial erosions Marginal infiltrates	Marginal infiltrates
Rosacea	Rare	Common

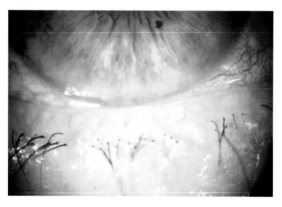

Figure 1.23   Anterior blepharitis with dystichiasis, polyosis, collarettes (epithelial aggregates around the base of lashes), anterior lid margin inflammation, and punctate corneal epithelial erosions at the inferior limbus

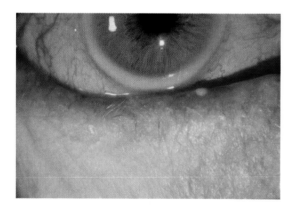

Figure 1.24   Posterior blepharitis with plugged and irregularly placed meibomian gland openings and rounded posterior lid margin with dilated vessels

Ectasia and irregular astigmatism

Irregularity in the thickness and tensile strength of the cornea leaves it prone to an irregular anterior corneal shape and warpage. It is convenient to think of the cornea as having a central optical zone of about 4 mm diameter (about the size of the pupil) and a peripheral non-optical zone comprising an annulus of about 4 mm across (Figure 1.25).

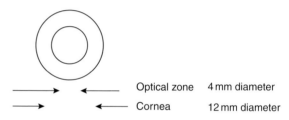

Figure 1.25   The cornea has an overall diameter of 12 mm and a central optical zone diameter of 4 mm

Irregularities of corneal thickness within the optical pathway affect the light path directly. Irregularities of the peripheral cornea affect the support of the optical zone, allowing it to warp and thus create irregularity of the anterior refracting surface of the central zone of the cornea. Irregularities of corneal thickness can be seen with the slit lamp. Irregularities in corneal refraction can be seen with the retinoscope.

Quantification of changes observed in the routine clinical examination

The shape of the anterior corneal surface can be quantified with keratometry and videokeratography. Keratometry is adequate for assessing the optical zone of the cornea ($4\,mm^2$) if the surface is regular and the astigmatism orthogonal. For more complicated corneas and when an assessment of a larger proportion of the cornea is required, videokeratography is preferable.

The process of diagnosis involves identifying the clinical features, understanding their pathobiological significance, and recognising a pattern of clinical disease by comparing the features of a patient with the patterns which experience has identified as recurring commonly. If a case does not fit with a commonly recurring pattern, the effective diagnostician will go back over the case, checking the findings and looking for unusual features.

Measurement of corneal thickness

Corneal hydration is carefully controlled under physiological conditions. This is necessary for transparency. Accumulation of water is associated with a loss of transparency and an increase in corneal thickness. The amount of water accumulated in the cornea is reflected in a proportional increase in corneal thickness.

Corneal thickness can be measured with either an optical or an ultrasonic pachymeter. Optical pachymetry has been used for many years but until recently was employed primarily for measuring central corneal thickness. Ultrasonic pachymetry has largely replaced conventional optical pachymetry. Although more expensive, ultrasonic pachymeters are easier to use, at least as accurate, and can be used to measure corneal thickness over the entire structure.

More recently, optical devices have been developed which can measure corneal thickness in the periphery and the axial zone of the cornea. They are an additional feature of advanced videokeratography devices.

Measurement of corneal curvature

The curvature of the anterior surface of the cornea is the most important refracting element in the optical system of the eye. Accurate measurement of corneal curvature is an important part of the clinical assessment of patients. Several techniques with varying levels of sophistication are used by clinicians to examine and measure anterior corneal curvature.

Retinoscopy

Retinoscopy is the oldest and simplest technique for measuring the refractive state of the eye and therefore of its most important element, the cornea. The clinician observes the movement of a small patch of illuminated retina and the refractive state is quantified by "neutralising" this movement with interposed lenses. Retinoscopy can only give broad warning of an abnormality of corneal shape and refraction but effective clinical ophthalmologists continue to rely on it as a cornerstone of general clinical assessment, despite the availability of automated apparatus for assessing the refractive state of the eye. Retinoscopy is a simple and inexpensive way of evaluating the refractive state of the eye and the clarity of the media and is more than adequate for diagnosing conditions such as subclinical keratoconus in patients with myopia.

Keratometry

The contribution of the most important refractive element of the optical system of the eye, the corneal surface, can be measured very easily and inexpensively with a keratometer. This instrument uses reflective optics to measure the curvature (or dioptic equivalent) of the maximum and minimum curvature in the optical zone. It is indispensable in the clinic, describing with considerable simplicity the refractive status of the cornea, but it does provide an oversimplified view of the corneal shape and dioptric power. Although this information is sufficient for the assessment of most refractive requirements for spectacles or contact lenses, it is not adequate when considering irregular deformities. More sophisticated apparatus is required for this purpose.

Videokeratography

Keratorefractive surgery has been a powerful stimulus for the development of sophisticated systems for mapping extensible corneal shape. Growing out of semiquantitative photokeratoscopy and based on the same principles of reflective optics, videokeratography involves relatively sophisticated systems for image capture, surface reconstruction, and data output.

Image capture involves projection of an image onto the surface of the cornea and capture of the reflected image with a digital video camera. Surface reconstruction depends on edge detection software and algorithms for calculating corneal shape (usually expressed as dioptric power) from the image analysis. Data output can be in several forms, such as data tables, colour coded curvature maps (Figure 1.26), or wire mesh models.

Despite obvious sophistication, modern instruments for determining corneal shape are based on a well known principle of reflection from the pseudospherical surface, or at least not from the entire surface, as the periphery is less curved than the central optical zone. Furthermore,

developments in videokeratography have revealed considerable irregular variation within individual corneas and from one person to another. There is a degree of symmetry from one eye to the contralateral eye but this is loose rather than rigid. There is also considerable variation from person to person. Corneal topographical maps have been likened to fingerprints, there being a similarity between apparently normal corneas but also distinct differences. Corneal topography may therefore be considered as another expression of the uniqueness of the individual.

Not only are maps of the corneal surface unique to the individual, they vary with time, even in people without any evidence of corneal disease. It is not clear whether this is always due to variations in the way the mapping apparatus is used, focus and centring being critical, or whether there are true variations in corneal shape. It is perhaps important to remember that

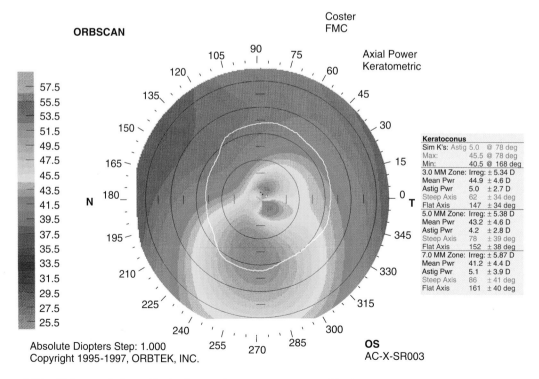

Figure 1.26   Colour coded graphical print-out from contemporary videokeratography device of a cornea affected by keratoconus

the shape determined by videokeratography is a measure of optical power, with true physical shape being inferred. In most situations, it is the corneal refractive power which is of interest and progress in videokeratography has developed parallel to keratorefractive surgery. There is a growing movement in refractive surgery which considers minor changes in corneal topography as important limitations on visual potential and amenability to surgery.

Trial of hard contact lens

It is not necessary to use sophisticated, and correspondingly expensive, videokeratography to determine the relevance of an irregular corneal surface. A time honoured and highly effective approach to this problem is to use a semi-rigid gas permeable lens to negate corneal surface irregularities. If irregularities in the shape, and therefore optical power, of the cornea are relevant to vision, a rigid contact lens will reveal the full visual potential or at least overcome any limitation imposed by the corneal shape (Figure 1.27).

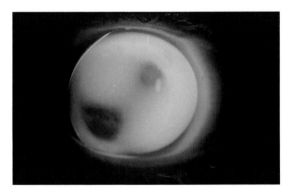

Figure 1.27 Fluorescein pattern under a rigid contact lens demonstrating an anterior corneal shape consistent with oblique regular astigmatism

Specular microscopy

Slit lamp examination of the cornea, using specular reflection, will reveal the endothelium but at relatively low magnification and in a very confined area.

A microscope developed by David Maurice in the 1960s has facilitated the observation and quantification of the corneal endothelium. It also uses specular reflection of light from the endothelium. Almost all light delivered to the cornea, around 99%, is transmitted to the aqueous humour. The remaining 1% is reflected off interfaces, one of the relevant interfaces being the endothelial monolayer. The endothelial cell membranes perpendicular to the curved plane of the endothelial monolayer forward scatter light, producing visible dark outlines to the cells and defining the endothelial mosaic.

The corneal endothelial microscope employs an applanating lens to flatten the cornea, which eliminates the air–tear interface, overcomes distortion due to corneal curvature, and immobilises the eye. Other features of the optical system of the microscope reduce reflections and widen the field of view. Magnification of up to 200 times can be achieved over a relatively large area (Figure 1.28).

Morphometric analysis is achieved digitally and contemporary devices will print out endothelial cell density, cell size, and variation in cell shape.

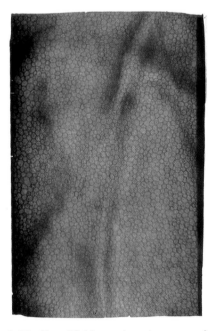

Figure 1.28 Broad field specular microscopy of normal corneal endothelium

The principal clinical use of endothelial specular microscopy is for serial measurement of endothelial cell density in response to surgical intervention. For this, it is an indispensable tool but for routine clinical matters the slit lamp is usually adequate.

Confocal microscopy

Contrast, and thereby resolution, of corneal microscopy can be increased by reducing scatter from above and below the plane of focus. This can be approached by reducing the field of view and using a point surface of light, with the focus of the illumination and viewing system the same or confocal.

This approach is well suited to the cornea and corneal confocal microscopes are available commercially. The high resolution of these systems allows *in vivo* examination of the cornea at a cellular level and digital z-axis reconstruction allows a three-dimensional examination of the cornea.

At this stage, these systems provide opportunities to improve clinical evaluation of the cornea, but they do not as yet have an established place in routine clinical practice.

Documenttaion of corneal signs

Clinical findings must be carefully recorded in the clinical notes. This can be done diagrammatically and various schemes have been proposed for doing this with varying levels of sophistication. A great deal of information can be recorded in a diagram of the cornea, particularly when colour coding is used, but clinicians generally carry a pen, not a box of coloured pencils. For this reason, it is appropriate to compromise and use a monochromatic system of lines (Figure 1.29).

In situations where it is important to observe change in the cornea, such as when managing inflammatory disorders, quantification of the signs is desirable. A picture may provide more information than a thousand words but one set of numbers can say more than a thousand pictures. A system for scoring inflammatory signs is set out in the section dealing with the treatment of inflammatory disease (Chapter 13, p. 144).

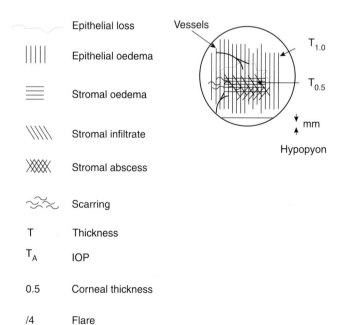

	Epithelial loss
	Epithelial oedema
	Stromal oedema
	Stromal infiltrate
	Stromal abscess
	Scarring
T	Thickness
T_A	IOP
0.5	Corneal thickness
/4	Flare
/4	Cells

Figure 1.29 A simple scheme for documenting corneal disease (Adapted from Bron AJ. *Br J Ophthalmol* 1973; **57**: 629–34.)

Development of the cornea

An understanding of corneal disease requires an appreciation of the way the cornea develops, its normal structure and function, and the pathological changes which can afflict it.

Embryology

After the lens vesicle separates from the surface ectoderm in the second month of gestation, three waves of neural crest cells move forward between the lens and the surface ectoderm. The first wave forms the corneal endothelium, the second the corneal stroma, and the third the stroma of the iris and the pupillary membrane.

The endothelial lining of the primitive anterior chamber is not achieved until the end of the fifth foetal month. Subsequently, the base of the iris moves posteriorly to expose the neural crest tissue which has developed into the trabecular meshwork. This posterior movement occurs because of differential rates of growth rather than by atrophy or cleavage, as was once thought. The posterior migration of the iris root continues during the first postnatal year (Figure 1.30).

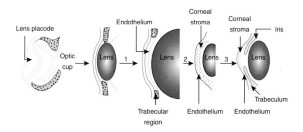

Figure 1.30 Development of the cornea (Reproduced with permission from Easty DL, Sparrow JM, eds. *Oxford Textbook of Ophthalmology*. Oxford: Oxford University Press, 1999.)

Developmental abnormalities of the cornea

Conditions developing as a consequence of abnormal neural crest migration and proliferation of differentiation are known collectively as neurocristopathies.

The relationship of developmental abnormalities of the anterior segment to each other and to embryological events was set out by Waring in 1975. This classification was proposed before the contribution of the neural crest to corneal development was recognised and when cleavage was thought to be the means by which the anterior chamber angle was created. Nevertheless, the classification does unify understanding of a number of unusual conditions. In recent years, some of the genetic influences on corneal development have been recognised (Box 1.1).

Homeobox gene and eye development

The homeobox gene PAX6, located on chromosome 11p13, is essential to the development of the eye. It plays an important role in the development of the lens and the organisation of the optic cup. PAX6 is expressed early in the optic pit and transcripts are later found in the developing eye vesicle, cornea, lens, and retina, suggesting that the gene may be involved in the regulation of some of the inductive events during the development of the eye. Both the inducing tissue (optic vesicle) and the induced tissue (overlying surface ectoderm) express PAX6. Individuals homozygous for mutations in PAX6 are anophthalmic and those who are heterozygous for such mutations have abnormalities in the cornea, iris, lens, and retina, including aniridia and Peter's anomaly.

The normal cornea at birth

At birth, the normal cornea is perfectly transparent, with a vertical diameter of 8 mm, a horizontal diameter of 10 mm, and anterior surface curvature of 7.1 mm.

Classification of congenital abnormalities

Congenital abnormalities of the cornea may affect the size and shape of the cornea, its curvature, and transparency. Such defects may occur in isolation, in association with

Box 1.1 *The findings in the anterior chamber cleavage syndrome. The table demonstrates the spectrum of anatomic combinations and the terms by which they are commonly known*

Posterior embryotoxon	Axenfeld's anomaly*	Rieger's anomaly*	Iridogonio-dysgenesis*	Posterior keratoconus	Peter's anomaly*†	Anterior chamber cleavage syndrome*
Prominent Schwalbe's ring	Prominent Schwalbe's ring	Prominent Schwalbe's ring				Prominent Schwalbe's ring
	Iris strands to Schwalbe's ring	Iris strands to Schwalbe's ring	Iris strands to Schwalbe's ring			Iris strands to Schwalbe's ring
		Hypoplasia anterior iris stroma	Hypoplasia anterior iris stroma			Hypoplasia anterior iris stroma
			Posterior corneal depression	Posterior corneal defect and leucoma	Posterior corneal defect and leucoma — Iris adhesions to leucoma margin — Lens apposition to leucoma	Posterior corneal defect and leucoma — Iris adhesions to leucoma margin — Lens apposition to leucoma

* May have developmental glaucoma.
† von Hippel's internal corneal ulcer, if inflammatory.

abnormalities in the eye remote from the cornea or in the face or other parts of the body (Table 1.2).

Anatomy of the adult cornea

The normal adult cornea measures 11–12 mm horizontally and 9–11 mm vertically (Figure 1.31). It is approximately 0.5 mm thick centrally and a little thicker than this, 0.65–0.70 mm, peripherally (Figure 1.32). The anterior radius of curvature is 7.5–8.0 mm centrally and flatter peripherally. The central 4 mm of the diameter of the cornea is considered to be the optical zone. This is the prepupillary cornea which is virtually spherical with a dioptric power of about 44 dioptres, about 75% of the dioptric power of the eye. The standard refractive index of the cornea is usually considered to be 1.3375.

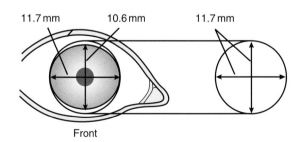

Figure 1.31   Dimensions of the normal adult cornea. Anterior and posterior view

Table 1.2 Features of the abnormalities in size and shape of the cornea

	Megalocornea	Microcornea	Corneal plana	Sclerocornea
Features	Corneal diameter 13–16.5 mm; bilateral, 90% male	Corneal diameter <10 mm	Corneal radius of curvature <7.84 mm; classically of similar curvature to sclera	Scleralisation of cornea; involves entire or peripheral cornea; bilateral
Inheritance	X-linked recessive	Dominant or recessive (less common)	Dominant or recessive	Sporadic, dominant or recessive
Ocular associations	Miosis; goniodysgenesis; cataract; ectopia lentis; glaucoma (not congenital)	Microphthalmos; nanophthalmos; hyperopia; glaucoma; cataracts; persistent hyperplastic primary vitreous; anterior segment dysgenesis; optic nerve hypoplasia	Hyperopia; microcornea; sclerocornea; cataracts; colobomas; glaucoma	Cornea plana
Systemic associations	Facial anomalies; craniosynostosis; dwarfism; mental retardation; Down's syndrome; Alport's syndrome; Marfan's syndrome	Fetal alcohol syndrome; Ehlers–Danlos syndrome; myotonic dystrophy; achondroplasia		

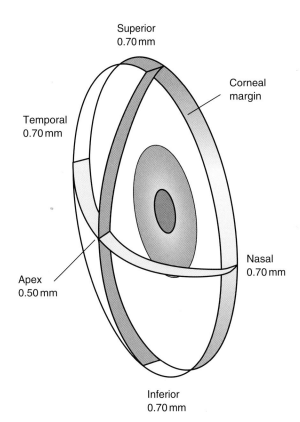

Superior
0.70 mm

Corneal margin

Temporal
0.70 mm

Nasal
0.70 mm

Apex
0.50 mm

Inferior
0.70 mm

Figure 1.32 The cornea is thicker at the periphery than it is centrally

Histology of the adult cornea

The histological structure of the cornea comprises five distinct layers (Figure 1.33):

- the epithelium
- Bowman's membrane
- the stroma
- Descemet's membrane
- the endothelium.

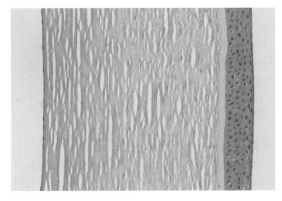

Figure 1.33 Histological section of the cornea showing epithelium, Bowman's layer, stroma, Descemet's membrane, and endothelium

21

Epithelium

The corneal epithelium comprises 5–6 layers of non-keratinising squamous epithelium. There is a basal monolayer of columnar cells, two or three layers of wing cells, and two or three layers of superficial non-keratinising squamous epithelial cells. Only the basal columnar cells show mitotic activity (Figure 1.34). Current opinion is that the corneal epithelial stem cells reside in the basal limbal epithelium and that the daughter cells migrate centrally and superficially with increasing differentiation and that the process of differentiation takes around 14 days under normal circumstances.

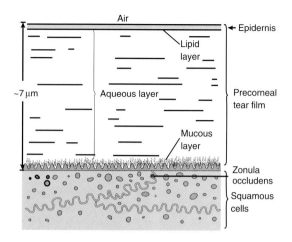

Figure 1.35 The precorneal tear film and the surface epithelium. The tear film is thought of as having lipid, aqueous, and mucinous layers, the mucin having an intimate relationship with the microvilli of the surface epithelium. Tight junctions between the superficial epithelial cells creates a barrier between the tear film and the epithelium

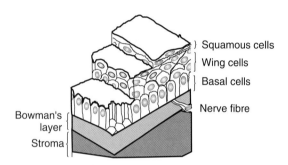

Figure 1.34 The cellular layers of the corneal epithelium, the surface microvilli, supporting Bowman's membrane, and a branching nerve fibre

Terminally differentiated corneal epithelial cells have a dense coat of microvilli which greatly increase the surface area of the cells and are evolved to carry out the active exchange of oxygen and nutrients between cells and tear fluid. These microvilli are also differentiated to hold mucus and thereby bind the precorneal tear film. Superficial cells are joined by desmosomes and tight junctional complexes, which have an important epithelial barrier function. Fully differentiated surface epithelial cells provide a complete barrier, preventing water from the tear film from entering the cornea (Figure 1.35).

Dendritic cells are also found in the peripheral corneal epithelium, but not centrally. They are the outposts of the immune system and are involved in antigen processing. The epithelium contributes about 10% of the corneal thickness.

Bowman's layer

Bowman's layer is at the interface between the epithelium and the stroma and comprises a compaction of collagen fibres (mainly types I and III) and proteoglycans. It is best considered as the anterior layer of stroma and has no regenerative powers.

Stroma

The stroma provides 90% of the corneal thickness. It comprises collagen, principally collagen I, and lesser amounts of type III, V, and VI glycosaminoglycans, mainly keratin sulphate. It also comprises chondroitin and dermatan sulphate, and cells, mainly corneal fibroblasts or keratocytes, which synthesise collagen and glycosaminoglycans, as well as collagen degradative enzymes, such as metalloproteases.

The collagen fibrils form approximately 300 distinct lamellae, each covering the entire area of the cornea parallel to the surface. Transparency of the cornea is attributed to the extremely regular spacing of the collagen fibrils which are separated by glycosaminoglycans, which are macromolecules with a role in maintaining even hydration of the stroma (Figure 1.36).

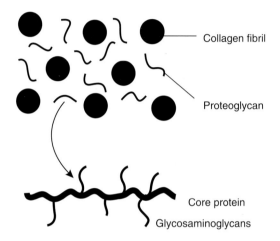

Figure 1.36 Proteoglycans have a core protein surrounded by glycosaminoglycans. Proteoglycans maintain a gel-like matrix between collagen fibrils

Keratocytes are arranged in a three-dimensional matrix, with their long processes insinuated between fibrils and making contact with other keratocytes with which they communicate through gap junctions (Figure 1.37).

Descemet's membrane

Descemet's membrane is the basement membrane of the corneal endothelium, although there are no anchoring structures between them. About 5–7 microns thick, it increases in thickness from about 2 to 3 microns at birth to 10 or 11 microns in old age. It comprises, principally, collagen type IV and laminin, but at least five types of collagen have been reported. The appearance can be abnormal in patients with endothelial disease, such as Fuchs' dystrophy.

Endothelium

The endothelium is a monolayer of hexagonal cells which have an important role in pumping water from the cornea and thus a major role in maintaining corneal transparency. Under normal circumstances, the hexagonal mosaic is remarkably regular. The important metabolic responsibilities of endothelial cells are reflected in their cytology; they have large nuclei with many well developed cytoplasmic organelles. In addition, there are well developed microvilli and marginal folds to increase the surface area of the cell and facilitate active pumping functions. Junctional complex structures, such as zonula occludens, macula occludens, and macula adherens, are abundant and endothelial cells communicate with each other through gap junctions (Figure 1.38).

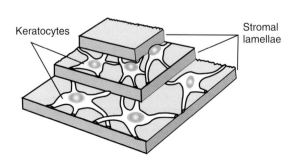

Figure 1.37 Keratocytes are found between the stromal lamellae. They have long processes which radiate out and contact other keratocytes

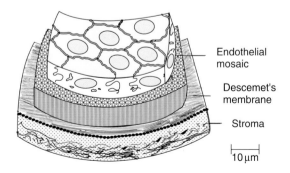

Figure 1.38 The corneal endothelium, a closely packed layer of hexagonal cells. Endothelial cells are adherent to each other and to Descemet's membrane

23

An important feature of endothelial cells is their inability to divide for purposes of repair. They are prone to injury from trauma, particularly surgery, and inflammation; loss of cells is covered by the remaining cells sliding and spreading out. In early adult life, the endothelial cell density is about 4000 to 5000 mm^2. This gradually reduces over the decades but may decrease dramatically after injury. Where the cell density is reduced below 1000 mm^2, the pumping function of the cornea is compromised and corneal oedema may result (Figure 1.39).

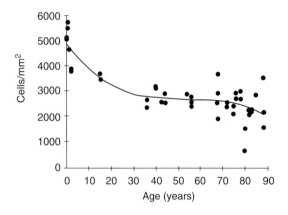

Figure 1.39 Endothelial cell density measured by specular microscopy. Density decreases with age (Reproduced with permission from Williams KK, Noe RL, Grossniklaus HE, Drews-Botsch C, Edelhauser HF. *Arch Ophthalmol* 1982; **110**: 1146.)

General pathology of the cornea

Corneal ulceration

Loss of the corneal epithelium is always of consequence because it is responsible for a number of critical functions. As the most important element in the refractive complex of the eye, it is a highly evolved surface epithelium which holds the tear film to create a perfectly shaped air–water interface. This interface is responsible for approximately 75% of the refractive power of the eye.

The epithelium also has an important protective function. The thin layer of cells is a buffer separating the delicate structures of the inner eye from microbes and toxins in the external environment. So important is this protective function that long-standing corneal ulceration is incompatible with the survival of the eye.

Corneal ulceration can be caused by physical trauma, exposure to chemicals, heat or infection (Figure 1.40). Epithelial loss can also occur spontaneously as a result of dystrophic conditions which weaken the usually effective adhesive mechanisms. Dystrophic epithelial instability may complicate a previous injury or may be part of an inherited dystrophic process. Spontaneous corneal ulceration may complicate anterior membrane dystrophy, Reis–Bücklers, granular, lattice and, less commonly, macular dystrophy.

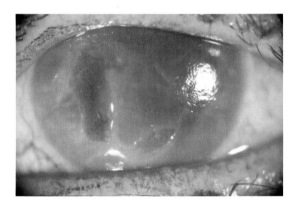

Figure 1.40 Extensive corneal ulceration due to herpes simplex virus and stained with rose bengal

Defective epithelium prone to ulceration can also result from pathology occurring primarily in other elements of the ecosystem of the outer eye. For example, severe tear deficiency may result in ulceration. So too may abnormalities in the limbal stem cells which are responsible for corneal epithelial cell replenishment.

Whatever the cause, corneal ulceration threatens the integrity of the eye. One of a number of sequelae of ulceration which can contribute to the threat is inflammation, a serious consequence.

Acute inflammation of the cornea

With sufficient stimulus, the cornea can mount an impressive acute inflammatory response. Common initiating factors are trauma, exposure to chemicals or toxins, and infection. Resolution, repair, and tissue damage with subsequent loss of vision may follow from the initial damage (Figure 1.41).

Acute corneal inflammation is characterised by dilation of vessels in the eye wall adjacent to the avascular cornea. Particularly at the limbus and iris, leakage of intravascular fluid to the extracellular space results in a proteinaceous aqueous which can be seen as flare and which contributes to corneal oedema. In addition, there is recruitment of inflammatory cells into the relatively acellular cornea from limbal vessels. Inflammatory cells also escape from dilated iris vessels and can be seen circulating in the aqueous humour. If present in large numbers, cells may settle in the anterior chamber to create a hypopyon. There is also impairment of normal metabolic functions at inflammatory sites; in the presence of inflammation, endothelial function is impaired, resulting in corneal oedema. Corneal oedema is a sensitive barometer of corneal inflammation. It is the first sign of inflammation when the cornea is challenged and the first sign to resolve when containing an inflammatory process. Acute inflammation can damage the cornea by a number of mechanisms (Figure 1.42).

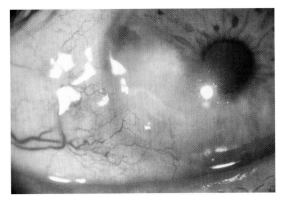

Figure 1.42 Corneal inflammation. Ulceration complicated by inflammation and abscess formation. Peripheral vascularisation suggests the development of chronicity

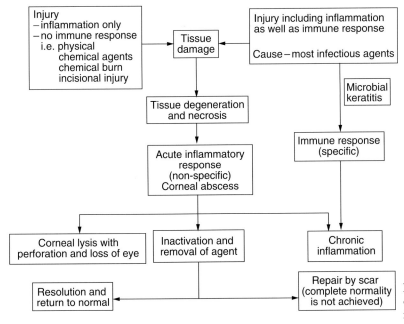

Figure 1.41 Various agents can cause corneal damage and induce inflammation

Stromal lysis

In the acute phase, intense inflammation may result in white cell recruitment sufficient to cause an abscess. The majority of inflammatory cells are polymorphs which contain within their lysozymes enzymes capable of disaggregating the cornea, causing tissue loss or stromal lysis. This process may occur very quickly, within hours of the onset of inflammation, and is the reason why corneal infection must be considered an ophthalmic emergency (Figure 1.43).

of limbal vessels, with neovascularisation, the formation of new vessels, and the proliferation and migration of fibroblasts followed by fibrosis. The new vessels are not functionally competent and leak intravascular contents into the corneal stroma. With chronic inflammation and neovascularisation there is often leakage of lipid from new vessels, resulting in lipid keratopathy. All these processes tend to interfere with the normal function of the cornea, thereby impairing vision (Figure 1.44).

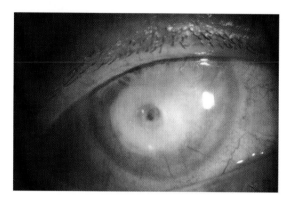

Figure 1.43 Acute inflammation of the cornea complicated by stromal lysis and perforation

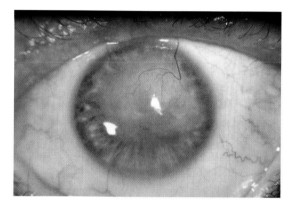

Figure 1.44 Chronic inflammation of the cornea with scarring, neovascularisation, and lipid deposition

In addition to acute corneolysis, there are other chronic sequelae of inflammation which are sight threatening.

Chronic inflammation

Chronic inflammation of the cornea may follow acute inflammation if the initiating factor persists or may occur as a primary condition without an identifiable acute phase. At a clinical level, chronic corneal inflammation is characterised by stromal oedema and cellular infiltration, scarring, and neovascularisation. At a histological level, chronicity is characterised by a change in the inflammatory cell population. The polymorph response of acute inflammation is replaced by a preponderance of lymphocytes, macrophages and, in some situations, giant cells. There is also "budding" of the endothelial cells

Chronic inflammation of the cornea can damage the eye by less direct mechanisms. In severe cases, inflammation of the cornea may involve adjacent structures. For example, the peripheral cornea, and the drainage structures contained therein, are often involved in keratitis. This results in secondary glaucoma.

Repair

Corneal repair is the desired outcome for all inflammatory episodes. The epithelium repairs by increasing cell division and slide, the stroma by fibrosis and the creation of matrix materials, and the endothelium by cell enlargement and slide.

Epithelial healing is necessary for the survival of the cornea and the eye. Failure of an epithelial defect to heal will expose the stroma to inappropriate hydration, provide a portal of entry for micro-organisms, and expose underlying structures to environmental toxins and foreign materials.

Stromal healing is required for tensile strength so that an appropriate corneal shape can be established and maintained (Figure 1.45).

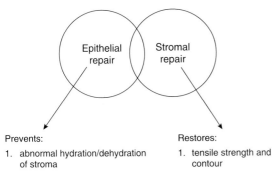

Prevents:
1. abnormal hydration/dehydration of stroma
2. microbial invasion
3. entry of toxins

Restores:
1. tensile strength and contour

Figure 1.45 Corneal repair is the most desirable outcome of corneal inflammation

Loss of corneal privilege

Another effect of corneal inflammation is the loss of immunological privilege. Several factors account for the way in which a normal cornea will tolerate allografts. These include the relative acellularity of normal cornea, the lack of blood vessels and lymphatics, and the constitutive expression of FasL by corneal cells. Inflammation erodes privilege by populating the stroma with cells derived from bone marrow (Figure 1.46). These can process antigen and initiate an immune response by creating blood vessels and lymphatics where they did not previously exist and by upregulation of MMC expression (Figure 1.47).

This erosion of corneal immune privilege by inflammation is a major clinical problem. Postinflammatory scarring is second only to cataract as a cause of blindness in the world. Millions of patients would benefit from a corneal transplant if their scarred cornea could be replaced by a normal transparent cornea. Unfortunately, in this group of patients allograft

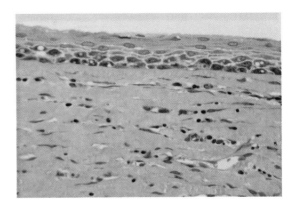

Figure 1.46 Corneas with chronic inflammation or corneas inflamed in the past carry increased numbers of cells derived from bone marrow. Transplants put into such a bed reject and the risk of rejection is proportional to the number of cells in the recipient cornea

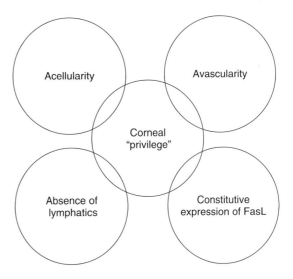

Figure 1.47 Factors contributing to corneal privilege

rejection leading to corneal graft failure is common for the reasons given above.

Oedema

Corneal oedema occurs as a consequence of inflammation, as well as for other reasons. Control of corneal hydration is largely due to endothelial function. When the corneal endothelium is compromised, corneal hydration increases. Endothelial cell function is adversely affected by trauma, inflammation, hypoxia, and elevated intraocular pressure or spontaneous breaks in Descemet's membrane, as occurs with keratoconus (Figure 1.48).

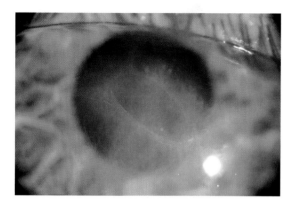

Figure 1.48 Corneal oedema due to focal endothelial deficiency resulting from spontaneous rupture of Descemet's membrane complicating keratoconus

Physical trauma may impact on the cornea immediately or some time later, even decades later. Direct trauma may be complicated immediately by oedema as is sometimes the case after blunt injuries. More often, oedema occurs much later as a consequence of endothelial cell loss. After an injury causing endothelial cell loss, repair occurs by cells enlarging and spreading and not by cell division. Even under normal conditions, there is a loss of endothelial cells over a lifetime but the rate of loss is not sufficient to leave the endothelium compromised unless there is a genetic predisposition, as in Fuchs' dystrophy. As a consequence of trauma, including intraocular surgery, endothelial cells may be lost at the time of injury but the subsequent loss of cells is above the normal rate. Corneal oedema may complicate corneal trauma years after the injury.

Oedema resulting from impairment of corneal endothelial function due to inflammation is seen in many clinical conditions. It is seen in its least complicated form where viral diseases, principally herpes simplex virus infection but also common childhood diseases such as mumps, chickenpox, rubella, measles, and glandular fever, cause central or sometimes eccentric corneal oedema, described as *disciform keratitis*.

Hypoxia compromising endothelial cell function is most commonly seen in contact lens wearers. Oedema occurs when oxygen transmission through a lens is insufficient for endothelial metabolic activity. This occurs when lenses with poor oxygen transmission are worn overnight. Under the closed-eye sleeping conditions, oxygen availability is decreased to a level where endothelial cell dysfunction occurs.

Oedema is initially confined to the stroma but as it progresses the epithelium becomes involved, with fluid accumulating in the epithelium to cause blisters, usually referred to as bullae. As the bullae rupture, epithelial nerve endings are exposed, resulting in considerable pain. Ulceration caused in this way is also a potential portal of entry for micro-organisms and the establishment of infection (Figure 1.49).

When oedema is chronic rather than acute, there is budding of endothelial cells in the limbal vasculature, leading to corneal neovascularisation.

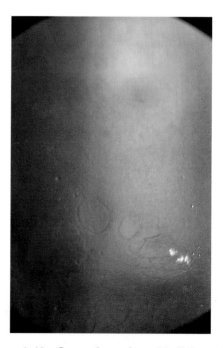

Figure 1.49 Stromal and epithelial oedema complicating prolonged overnight contact lens wear. Rupture of epithelial bullae results in ulceration and increased risk of infection

This is the mechanism of corneal vascularisation seen in contact lens wearers.

Corneal oedema is invariably associated with decreased vision. In the oedematous cornea, the spatial arrangement of the collagen fibrils of the stroma is disturbed so that transparency is lost. Acuity is reduced and light is dispersed so that point sources of light are spread on the retina and haloes are seen around lights.

Corneal deposits

Material may be deposited in the cornea. This may be abnormal molecular products as occurs in metabolic disorders, such as inherited storage diseases, or as occurs in inherited corneal dystrophies. Ionic material may be held in the cornea, such as calcium bound to Bowman's membrane in band keratopathy (Figure 1.50), copper bound to Descemet's membrane in Wilson's disease (Figure 1.51), or iron bound to the epithelium around the base of a conical cornea (Figure 1.52). Large molecules, such as proteins, can accumulate in the stroma if blood levels are high, as occurs with monoclonal gammopathies (Figure 1.53). Lipid accumulation is common when the normally avascular cornea develops new blood vessels and lipid can also accumulate in the cornea as a complication of hyperlipidaemia (Figure 1.54).

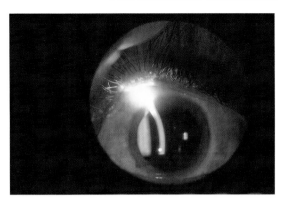

Figure 1.51 Copper bound to peripheral Descemet's membrane in Wilson's disease

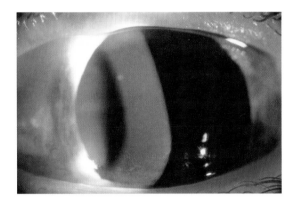

Figure 1.52 Iron bound to the epithelium around the base of a conical cornea

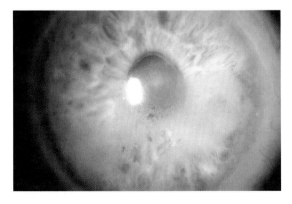

Figure 1.50 Band keratopathy. Calcium deposition in Bowman's membrane

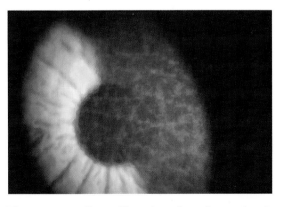

Figure 1.53 Crystalline deposits of proteins in the corneal stroma in a patient with monoclonal gammopathy

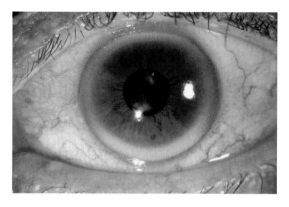

Figure 1.54 Arcus senilis. Deposition of lipid in the peripheral corneal stroma in a patient with hyperlipidaemia

Ectasia

Ectasia is a term used to describe weakening of the cornea so that its tensile strength is reduced. Keratoconus in its various clinical manifestations is the result of this process. The weakening can be attributed to decreased corneal thickness, an abnormality of collagen, or abnormal ground substance. As a consequence the intraocular pressure protrudes the cornea in a conical shape. If the cornea cannot hold an appropriate shape for refraction, vision is impaired. In keratoconus, the tensile strength of the cornea cannot withstand the intraocular pressure and a conical protrusion of the cornea occurs (Figure 1.55).

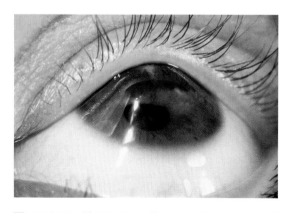

Figure 1.55 Keratoconus. Decreased tensile strength of the cornea results in conical protrusion

Epithelial disorders

The epithelium is the most active layer of the cornea in relation to cell turnover. This is reflected in the propensity of the corneal epithelium to exhibit abnormalities of cell division and differentiation. Hyperplasia, metaplasia, dysplasia, and neoplasia all occur. Fortunately, minor abnormalities of growth and differentiation are common and more serious abnormalities, such as neoplasia, are rare (Figure 1.56).

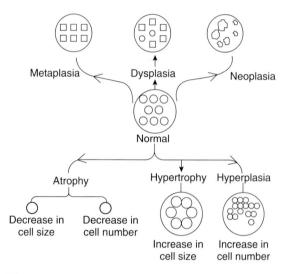

Figure 1.56 Disorders of cell growth and differentiation which occur in the corneal epithelium

Hyperplasia

Epithelial hyperplasia of the cornea occurs when the cornea develops an unusual shape, as occurs after corneal surgery and over areas of stromal inflammation. The proliferation of morphological normal epithelium tends to even up the surface of the cornea.

Metaplasia

Epithelial metaplasia of the cornea is also common. The transition of the stratified corneal epithelium usually occurs under chronic stress conditions, such as long term irritation, or when the tear film is deficient. Under such circumstances, the corneal epithelium tends to become more squamous and tends, with particularly stressful conditions, to become keratinised.

Dysplasia

Epithelial dysplasia of the cornea, where there is disordered growth which can be considered the precursor of malignancy, occurs less frequently than the above. Almost invariably the dysplastic process begins at the limbus and the area of dysplastic epithelium can be seen clinically. No cause is apparent.

Neoplasia

Neoplasia of the corneal epithelium may occur in an area of dysplasia or may occur independently. In either case, the process usually begins at the limbus. The malignant transformation of the epithelium may be limited by the basement membrane (carcinoma *in situ*) or the process may be more extensive and breach the basement membrane (invasive squamous cell carcinoma). Sometimes all three entities, dysplasia, carcinoma *in situ* and invasive carcinoma, can be seen in the same cornea.

Benign papillomata

Not all tumours of the cornea and limbus are malignant. Benign papillomata, which also occur at the limbus, are due to infection with papilloma virus. In these lesions, the normal arrangement of epithelium to connective tissue is seen and the arrangement of blood vessels is obvious, but with normal structures. Malignant transformation of these tumours is rare.

Control of corneal epithelial differentiation

Differentiation of epithelial cells is influenced by various factors. The first requirement for appropriate differentiation is an appropriate stem cell. Corneal epithelial stem cells reside in the limbal region in the palisades of Vogt. Under physiological conditions, a cell in its local environment is subject to numerous signals. Although current knowledge is incomplete, some

influences have been identified. Soluble factors and cellular, matrix and neuronal elements influence the development of appropriately differentiated corneal epithelial cells from limbal stem cells (Figure 1.57).

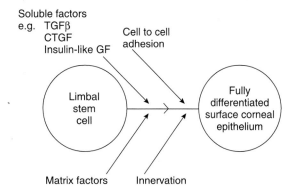

Figure 1.57 Normal growth and full differentiation of corneal epithelium requires soluble factors, matrix factors, cell to cell communication, and normal innervation

Soluble factors, such as epithelial growth factor, TGFβ, connective tissue growth factor, and insulin-like growth factor, are produced by corneal tissues and influence growth and differentiation of corneal cells. This effect may be direct on cells or via the matrix.

The matrix, which has a bearing on epithelial differentiation, is composed of collagen and the related macromolecules, including the glycosaminoglycans. At the very least, the matrix acts as a binder for soluble factors which influence growth and differentiation. The matrix also contains molecules which act as adhesion mechanisms and bind epithelial cells. Stem cells are particularly dependent on the microniche provided by the matrix to maintain their position and to divide and differentiate. Adhesion to the matrix is by integrins, a family of integral cell membrane proteins which bind cells to other cells and to matrix elements.

Cell to cell adhesion and communication depend on integrins. Close approximation of cells and active communication is also important in cell differentiation. Adjacent cells tend to achieve similar directions in differentiation, even with non-infective conditions. This accounts for the focal changes seen in many abnormalities of the corneal epithelium, such as punctate keratopathy.

Innervation is also important. It is well known that corneal sensory nerves affect corneal growth and repair in addition to their role in perception. Denervation of the cornea results, at worst, in neurotrophic ulceration and, at best, in metaplasia. There is not at present a clear explanation of the non-nociceptive role of corneal sensory nerves, but it is known that growth, differentiation, and migration of corneal epithelial cells *in vitro* are influenced by the neuropeptide substance P and insulin-like growth factor.

Metaplasia of corneal epithelium

Metaplasia is a general term describing aberrant epithelial differentiation. Full differentiation of the corneal epithelium is essential for normal corneal function. Two aspects of corneal differentiation are critical for normal function. First, the superficial surfaces of fully differentiated epithelial cells have characteristic brush borders due to microvilli projecting from their surface; it is these structures which hold the mucus and support the precorneal tear film. Second, fully differentiated epithelial cells have tight occluding junctions with neighbouring cells. The less terminally differentiated basal cells also have effective adhesion with the underlying basement membrane.

Failure to fully differentiate and achieve microvilli, occlusive cellular connections, and basal cell adherence to the basement membrane has serious consequences (Figure 1.58).

Degenerative disorders of the cornea

Degenerative conditions also occur in the cornea. As it is an exposed mucosal surface, the ocular surface is affected by climatic conditions, in particular by sunlight. At the limbus, exposure to ultraviolet light over a long

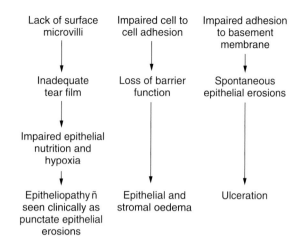

Figure 1.58 Failure of corneal epithelium to achieve full differentiation has serious clinical consequences

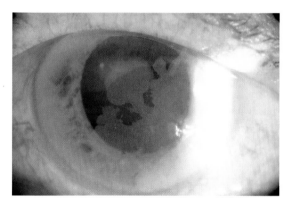

Figure 1.59 Dysplasia and carcinoma *in situ* in the corneal epithelium

period can produce similar changes to those of actinic elastosis of the skin. Degenerative changes are found in the subepithelial region, with loss of elastin fibrils and accumulation of amorphous agranular material. There are also active fibroblasts and the overlying epithelium may be normal, atrophic, or hyperplastic. Squamous metaplasia, with or without keratinisation, dysplasia (Figure 1.59) or even carcinoma *in situ* may be associated but invasive malignancy is most uncommon. Minor lesions confined to the limbal conjunctiva are termed *pinguecula* (Figure 1.60). Larger lesions growing into the cornea and with a fibrotic subepithelial element are called *pterygia* (Figure 1.61).

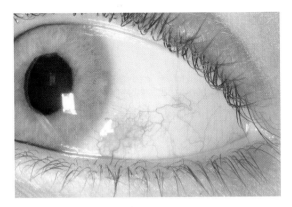

Figure 1.60 Pingueculum at the lower temporal limbus

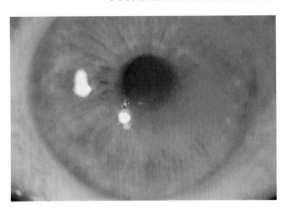

Figure 1.62 Band keratopathy. Calcium is bound to Bowman's membrane

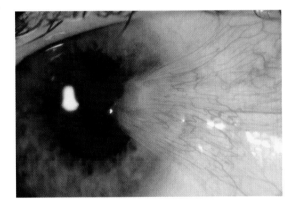

Figure 1.61 Pterygium

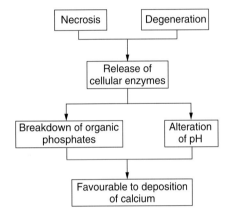

Figure 1.63 Cellular mechanisms favouring calcium deposition in degenerative and dystrophic conditions

Calcification

Bowman's membrane is prone to calcification, a condition termed *band keratopathy*. For some reason, calcium is attracted to and fixed in the macromolecules of the structure (Figure 1.62). Perhaps the cause is similar to that which results in the deposition of copper in Descemet's membrane in patients with Wilson's disease, a situation where the molecular structure of the membrane provides a binding site for the copper ion.

Deposition of calcium in Bowman's membrane occurs in two circumstances: dystrophic calcification and metastatic calcification.

Calcification is a feature of chronic inflammatory and degenerative disorders, chronic ocular inflammation being the most common cause of band keratopathy (Figure 1.63). Less

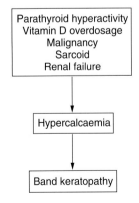

Figure 1.64 Causes of hypercalcaemia which may lead to band keratopathy

commonly, band keratopathy is due to metastatic calcification as a complication of increased blood calcium (Figure 1.64).

Major patterns of corneal disease

Even though a vast array of pathological processes may occur in the cornea, a relatively small number of distinct patterns of clinical disease present to the clinician. Some patterns occur frequently and within each of the commonly recurring patterns, there are recognisable variations. What constitutes a "major pattern of corneal disease" is somewhat arbitrary, but it is nevertheless helpful to recognise common groups of disorders to assist in the development of a disciplined approach to diagnosis.

In terms of frequency of presentation, two groups of corneal disease are particularly important. First, inflammatory disorders of the external eye and the anterior segment are particularly common. Inflammatory conditions in and around the cornea are particularly threatening and deserve priority, in both discussion and action. Second, trauma is important for much the same reason. The cornea, as the exposed element of the eye wall, is prone to trauma and since it has an important protective role, anything which threatens or breaches it poses a threat to vision.

Other patterns occur less frequently but are very distinctive. Although less common, they are important because they may affect vision or be part of a systemic disorder which may be threatening to a patient's general health.

When considering the clinical conditions which affect the cornea, it is appropriate to start with the "major patterns of corneal disease" and to develop strategies for diagnosing and treating the specific clinical entities within the major groups. Major patterns of corneal disease fall into three groups: conditions associated with inflammation; conditions associated with trauma; and non-inflammatory conditions. The subsequent sections of this book are based on these groupings.

Further reading

Bahn CF, Falls HF, Varley GA et al. Classification of corneal endothelial disorders based on neural crest origin. Ophthalmology 1984; **91**: 558–63.

Beebe DC. Homeobox genes and vertebrate eye development. Invest Ophthalmol Vis Sci 1994; **35**: 2897–900.

Benedek GB. Theory of transparency of the eye. Appl Optics 1971; **10**: 459.

Bron AJ, Seal DV. The defences of the ocular surface. Trans Ophthalmol Soc UK 1986; **105**: 18.

Coats G. Small superficial opaque white rings in the cornea. Trans Ophthalmol Soc UK 1912; **32**: 53.

Cogan DG, Albright F, Bartter FC. Hypercalcemia and band keratopathy. Arch Ophthalmol 1948; **40**: 624.

Dikstein S, Maurice DM. The metabolic basis to the fluid pump in the cornea. J Physiol 1972; **221**: 29.

Dohlman C. The function of the corneal epithelium in health and disease. Invest Ophthalmol 1971; **10**: 383.

Dougherty DM, Silvany RE, Meyer DR. The role of tetracycline in chronic blepharitis: inhibition of lipase production in staphylococci. Invest Ophthalmol Vis Sci 1991; **32**: 2970.

Fogle JA, Kenyon KR, Stark WJ et al. Defective epithelial adhesion in anterior corneal dystrophy. Am J Ophthalmol 1975; **79**: 925.

Gass JD. The iron lines of the superficial cornea: Hudson-Stähle line, Stocker's line, and Fleischer's ring. Arch Ophthalmol 1964; **71**: 348.

Hogan MJ, Alvarado JA, Weddell E. Histology of the Human Eye. Philadelphia: WB Saunders, 1971.

Johnston MC, Noden DM, Hazelton RD, Coulombre JL, Coulombre AJ. Origins of avian ocular and periocular tissues. Exp Eye Res 1979; **29**: 27–43.

Khodadoust AA, Silverstein AM, Kenyon KR et al. Adhesion of regenerating corneal epithelium. The role of basement membrane. Am J Ophthalmol 1968; **65**: 339.

Kruse FE. Stem cells and corneal epithelial regeneration. Eye 1994; **8**: 170–83.

Marshall GE, Konstas AGP, Lee WR. Collagens in ocular tissues. Br J Ophthalmol 1993; **77**: 515–24.

Maurice DM. The location of the fluid pump in the cornea. J Physiol 1972; **221**: 43.

Robert L, Jungua S, Moczar M. Structural glycoproteins of the intercellular matrix. Front Matrix Biol 1976; **3**: 113.

Smith GTH, Taylor HR. Epidemiology of corneal blindness in developing countries. Refract Corneal Surg 1991; 7: 436–9.

Waring GO, Rodrigues MM, Laibson PR. Anterior chamber cleavage syndrome: a stepladder classification. Surv Ophthalmol 1975; **20**: 3–27.

The following figures in this chapter were produced with kind permission from: Oyster CW. The Human Eye: Structure and Function. Sunderland, MA: Sinauer Associates Inc., 1999. 1.7a, 1.8a, 1.9a, 1.10, 1.32, 1.34, 1.35, 1.37, 1.38.

2 The cornea and inflammation: diagnosing the red eye

About half the patients presenting for emergency eye care have ocular inflammation (Figure 2.1). Many of these patients have corneal diseases or other conditions which threaten the cornea and vision. Clinicians require an effective strategy for diagnosing patients with a red eye. The strategy employed must give priority to finding the most threatening conditions, particularly the treatable ones, and not simply to considering the conditions that are most likely in the statistical sense. It is also important that the approach be simple and take into account the observation that in pattern recognition we consider only three or four variables at a time.

In looking for the major patterns of clinical disease in patients presenting with ocular inflammation, there are four major questions to be addressed.

Is the patient a contact lens wearer?

If contact lenses are worn, they must be removed before the evaluation proceeds. There are various forms of ocular inflammatory disease that are specific to contact lens wearers (for example, contact lens ulceration which may or may not be infected, hypoxia, epithelial erosion, giant papillary conjunctivitis, and sensitivity to lens maintenance solutions) (Figure 2.2). The patient needs to be assessed with this in mind but only after the general assessment has been completed. These entities are considered in a subsequent section.

Patients who wear contact lenses can develop inflammation as a consequence of contact lens wear, but they are as likely as anyone else to develop other inflammatory conditions not related to contact lens wear. A more detailed description of the corneal complications of contact lenses is set out in Chapter 5.

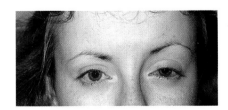

Figure 2.1 A patient presenting with ocular inflammation. This is one of the most frequent reasons for patients to present to an ophthalmologist

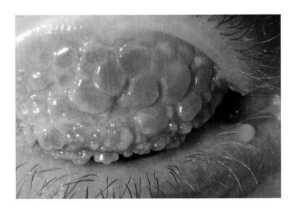

Figure 2.2 Conjunctivitis in a contact lens wearer. The conjunctival reaction with large papillae occurs principally in soft lens wearers

35

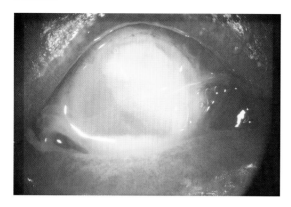

Figure 2.3 Corneal ulceration. Along with angle closure glaucoma, the most sight threatening cause of a red eye

Is the cornea ulcerated?

Corneal ulceration is a serious threat to the eye. If the ulcer is infected, the threat is acute. An untreated infected ulcer can destroy the cornea in less than 24 hours (Figure 2.3).

Corneal ulceration may take many forms. For example, the epithelial defect may be due to trauma or have arisen as a spontaneous erosion, it may be associated with infection, or due to denervation of the cornea, drug toxicity, allergy, or lid disease. It is usually possible to distinguish the various forms of ulceration from the clinical assessment.

It is important to know how long the patient has been symptomatic and whether there has been any previous eye disease. The duration of symptoms reflects the cadence of the process. In the absence of precipitating trauma, a brief period between the onset of symptoms and the presence of significant clinical disease indicates a threatening situation, such as an infection. Corneal infection can destroy an eye within hours.

A history of previous disease in the affected eye is also important. Corneal infection rarely occurs in eyes which do not have existing or pre-existing corneal disease. Herpetic keratitis is more likely than not to be recurrent.

It is necessary to examine the entire outer eye and not just the cornea, as some forms of ulceration are associated with specific conditions in the conjunctiva and lids. For example, "shield ulcers"; are associated with allergic conjunctivitis and corneal ulceration is often the result of lid disease that projects the lashes back against the cornea.

Two other aspects of the clinical pattern demand close examination: the state of the underlying stroma and the morphology of the ulcer. If there is oedema or infiltration of the underlying corneal stroma with inflammatory cells, it is very likely that there is an infective element involved. Under these circumstances, it is prudent to assume that the cornea is infected until proven otherwise.

It is important to look at the morphology of the ulcer. In particular, to look at the size and shape of the epithelial defect and then to look at the details of the ulcer margin. Some ulcers have a characteristic size and shape; for example, dendritic or geographic ulcers due to herpes simplex virus. Dendritic patterns also occur on the cornea for other reasons. They may occur in the process of epithelial healing of an erosion or abrasion or with the keratitis which develops with herpes zoster ophthalmicus. In each of these cases, close examination of the ulcer morphology and, in particular, the epithelial edge will distinguish the various entities. The lesions of herpes zoster ophthalmicus are raised and are in fact not ulcers at all but mucus plaques on the surface of the epithelium. The two entities are best differentiated by staining the cornea with rose bengal and fluorescein. With dendritic ulcers, the epithelial edge stains with rose bengal and the exposed stroma stains with fluorescein. With mucus plaques, the reverse happens – the mucus stains with rose bengal and the fluorescein pools around the edge.

It is necessary to examine the non-ulcerated areas of the affected eye and the contralateral eye. Spontaneous corneal erosions occur in eyes which have been previously traumatised or which are predisposed by an anterior membrane dystrophy. It should be possible to see evidence to support each of these possibilities, but to do so it is necessary to examine both eyes.

It is important to assess the corneal innervation by examining the corneal reflex. Denervation is often complicated by corneal ulceration. When examining patients with corneal disease, the corneal reflex should be checked before instilling any drops, such as mydriatics or local anaesthetic agents for measuring the intraocular pressure. If the stroma is inflamed, as evidenced by oedema or cellular infiltration, it is mandatory to assume that the cornea is infected until proven otherwise. One should be particularly suspicious if the eye is predisposed to infection by existing pathology, usually pre-existing epithelial disease, a brief history of accelerating symptoms, and a brisk inflammatory reaction in the anterior chamber rather than in the stroma. This clinical picture can also result from infection with herpes simplex virus, particularly when there has been previous recurrent herpetic disease. Although serious, this condition is not as threatening as bacterial keratitis and therefore is given lower priority in the diagnostic process. Bacterial infection can complicate herpetic disease and whenever the stroma is inflamed under an ulcer it is necessary to assume the worst and to consider the patient as having an infected cornea, regardless of whether there has been previous herpetic keratitis.

If a patient with an inflamed eye does not have a corneal ulcer, it is necessary to proceed with further questions. A more detailed discussion of corneal ulceration follows in Chapter 3.

Is there intraocular inflammation?

Intraocular inflammation may account for someone presenting with a red eye. There are various causes and the consequences of some of them are grave. Early identification of the cause of the inflammation is mandatory. These conditions are important in the context of corneal disease because they may present to the corneal surface and may have prominent corneal signs. The two most threatening conditions presenting with intraocular inflammation are angle closure glaucoma and uveitis.

Angle closure glaucoma

This is a medical emergency that threatens sight. It tends to occur in the elderly with large crystalline lenses and hypermetropes with small eyes. The intraocular pressure may reach a level sufficient to infarct the iris and ciliary body; this accounts for the inflammatory reaction in the anterior chamber. The high intraocular pressure may also impair the endothelial pump, resulting in corneal oedema which may suggest a primary disease of the cornea, especially if the ciliary body has also been damaged by the high pressure and the intraocular pressure has fallen to normal or below (Figure 2.4).

Uveitis

This intraocular inflammation may arise *de novo* and cause a patient to present with a

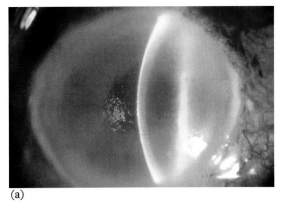

(a)

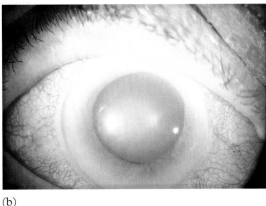

(b)

Figure 2.4 (a) Angle closure glaucoma tends to occur in older patients who often have hypermetropia and cataract. (b) The anterior chamber is shallow and the pupil distorted by ischaemia

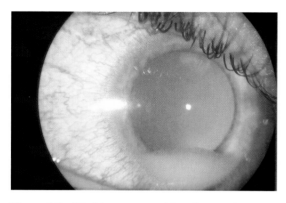

Figure 2.5 Uveitis presents with pain, a red eye and evidence of intraocular inflammation

painful red eye. Corneal signs may be a prominent feature of the clinical presentation. There are usually aggregations of inflammatory cells on the endothelial surface of the cornea and, if the eye is significantly inflamed, the endothelial pump may be compromised and the cornea oedematous (Figure 2.5).

The inflammatory signs in the anterior chamber are the classic signs of inflammation but perhaps seen more obviously than in any other clinical situation. Inflammatory cells can be seen circulating in the aqueous humour and aggregating on the posterior surface of the cornea; blood vessels in the iris become dilated and easily visible; and the loss of proteins from the vessels to the anterior chamber creates visible flare when a light is projected through the normally optically clear aqueous humour. Blood vessels in surrounding vascular tissues, such as the conjunctiva, episclera and sclera, also dilate, making the eye red and the vessels over the ciliary body particularly flushed to create a "ciliary flush".

Many ocular and systemic conditions develop intraocular inflammation. Although an account of these conditions is beyond the scope of this discussion, some have specific corneal manifestations. For example, ocular disorders, such as herpes simplex virus infection, may present with uveitis as the initial clinical event or as recurrent disease when earlier episodes have affected the cornea. Systemic inflammatory conditions can also affect intraocular tissues and the eye wall, including the cornea. As a general rule, systemic inflammatory diseases which are rheumatoid factor positive, such as rheumatoid arthritis, primarily affect the eye wall and those that are rheumatoid factor negative, such as HLA B27 associated conditions, primarily affect the uvea. A few, such as systemic lupus erythematosus, may be associated with both intraocular and eye wall inflammation but this is unusual. Chronic intraocular inflammation may result in secondary inflammation such as band keratopathy which is the deposition of calcium in Bowman's membrane. This is a common event in patients with juvenile arthritis and uveitis. Much less common is damage to the corneal endothelium or deposition of amyloid in the cornea as a consequence of chronic ocular inflammation.

If there is no corneal ulcer and no intraocular inflammation, the eye wall must be involved. This generates the fourth question.

Where is the focus of eye wall inflammation?

The eye wall is composed of the cornea, sclera, episclera, and conjunctiva. Each of these entities is subject to specific inflammatory disorders. Although keratitis, scleritis, episcleritis, and conjunctivitis occur as distinct entities, there is inevitably some overlap. When one of the tissues in the eye wall is inflamed there is usually some inflammation in adjacent tissues.

Keratitis

Keratitis occurs in many forms and can be due to multiple causes. Inflammation may be focused in the stroma, epithelium, or endothelium. Inflammation confined to the stroma is described as interstitial keratitis. Although originally used by Hutchinson in the 1850s to describe stromal keratitis associated with syphilis, in most societies today interstitial keratitis is due to herpes simplex virus infection but can be associated with herpes zoster ophthalmicus or a number of systemic inflammatory diseases, such as polyarteritis nodosa, Wegener's disease or rheumatoid arthritis. With these systemic inflammatory disorders, the inflammation tends to occur in the peripheral stroma which is a consequence of the vascular contribution to the peripheral cornea.

Epithelial keratitis also takes many forms, including punctate, filamentary, and ulcerative keratitis. These conditions are common and will be described in detail in the section on superficial keratopathy.

Endothelial keratitis is less common and tends to manifest with corneal oedema in the region of the compromised endothelium. This occurs with herpes simplex virus infection and with various other common systemic viral diseases. The clinical manifestation is a disc of corneal stromal oedema with a variable amount of inflammatory cell infiltrate, hence the clinical description of disciform keratitis.

Episcleritis

Episcleritis, inflammation of the episcleral connection tissue, is a common, usually self-limiting condition. It can be distinguished from conjunctivitis and scleritis on clinical grounds. There is no discharge, as occurs in conjunctivitis, and the pattern of infection is that of the episcleral vessels, not the conjunctival vessels or the larger, more sinusoidal scleral vessels. The pattern of inflammation is usually diffuse but may be nodular. It is often recurrent, recurring every few months, with each attack lasting for 7–10 days.

Scleritis

Scleritis is common and results in a red inflamed eye. The pain is usually dull rather than sharp and tends to be exacerbated by eye movements. The vessels in the area of inflamed sclera are large sinusoidal veins that tend to give the sclera a plum colour, especially when viewed under natural light, away from the slit lamp. The sclera may be diffusely or focally affected and the

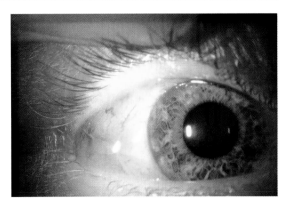

Figure 2.6   Scleritis. Inflammation may be confined to the sclera or may involve the contiguous corneal stroma

inflammation may involve the anterior or posterior sclera. When the posterior sclera is involved there may be few external signs of inflammation and the condition may present with symptoms suggestive of a retinal disorder. Inflammation in scleritis may be mild or severe (Figure 2.6). More severe cases present with intensely inflamed nodules and the inflammation may be so severe as to be necrotising and lead to perforation. Scleritis may also involve the contiguous cornea, hence the term *sclerokeratitis*.

Conjunctivitis

Conjunctivitis is perhaps the most common reason for patients presenting with an inflamed eye. There are many forms of conjunctivitis but they can usually be distinguished from one another with a sound clinical assessment. Conjunctivitis is usually bilateral, though not necessarily symmetrical, and usually produces a discharge the nature of which varies with the cause. Bacterial infection tends to produce a purulent discharge, viral infection a watery discharge, and allergic conjunctivitis can result in excessive mucus secretion (Figure 2.7).

With time, the conjunctiva may display secondary or responsive changes as part of the pattern of clinical expression. Infection with viruses or chlamydia will, after a few days, produce a follicular response. Allergic conditions, including

39

vernal conjunctivitis and conjunctivitis related to contact lens use, can result in the development of papillae.

Systemic inflammatory disorders may also be responsible for conjunctivitis. Conjunctivitis is part of both Reiter's disease and Behçet's disease.

Some forms of conjunctivitis are associated with corneal inflammation, hence the term *keratoconjunctivitis*. Adenoviral, chlamydial, and herpes simplex virus conjunctivitis can all produce punctate superficial keratitis. Allergic conjunctivitis can cause the deposition of mucus plaques on the cornea which can be so tightly adherent to the underlying corneal epithelium that it creates filaments, which may lead to corneal ulceration. If the mucus impacts on the stromal bed of a corneal ulcer the plaque can become thick and resemble a shield, hence the term *shield ulcer*.

Mucus adherence to the corneal epithelium occurs in some other conjunctival conditions. For example, the superior bulbar conjunctiva may become inflamed where the superior tarsal conjunctiva rubs against the globe during blinking. The upper corneal epithelium also becomes involved in the process, with filament formation. This condition is described as *superior limbic keratoconjunctivitis*.

More chronic conditions can also affect the conjunctiva and the cornea. Chlamydial infection is the cause of trachoma, which remains a blinding scourge in some parts of the world. This chronic form of conjunctivitis results in subepithelial scarring which distorts and contorts the eyelids, bringing the lashes back into contact with the globe and resulting in recurrent ulceration and scarring, leading to blindness in severe prolonged cases. In addition to scarring, the glandular elements in the conjunctiva are destroyed, resulting in a deficiency in the tear film which also contributes to pathological changes in the cornea. The same process occurs in systemic scarring diseases, such as Stevens–Johnson syndrome, pemphigoid and similar conditions, such as linear IgA disease, conditions in which the initiating events are not yet understood. These too can have devastating effects on vision as a consequence of the corneal complications of conjunctival disease.

Ocular inflammation is a common reason for patients presenting to the ophthalmologist. It is essential that a methodical search be made for the underlying cause along the lines suggested above and summarised in Figure 2.8.

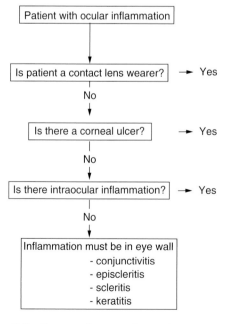

Figure 2.8   Strategy for assessing patients presenting with ocular inflammation

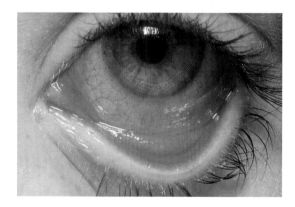

Figure 2.7   Conjunctivitis. Inflammation is confined to the conjunctiva and usually produces a discharge, and some result in changes in the corneal epithelium

3 Corneal ulceration

Corneal ulceration is a serious problem. As an essential element of the cornea and the eye, the corneal epithelium is differentiated to hold the precorneal tear film which is vital for vision and the nutrition and oxygenation of the superficial cornea. In addition, the epithelium is a tight barrier protecting the underlying cornea from imbibing water from the tear film and chemicals and toxins from the environment. Perhaps even more important is the role of the epithelium in protecting the eye from infection. It is an impenetrable barrier to most organisms.

As important as it is to vision, the corneal epithelium is vulnerable and prone to trauma, infection, and to numerous factors influencing the growth and differentiation of epithelial cells. There are many causes of corneal ulceration.

It is important to recognise corneal ulceration and to identify the underlying cause promptly if the blinding sequelae are to be avoided. Corneal ulceration is invariably complicated by loss of vision and even loss of the eye if epithelial healing does not occur. The major threats posed by corneal ulceration are infection, which can occur at any point in the history of an ulcer, and stromal scarring, which can complicate the associated acute or chronic stromal inflammation.

Causes of corneal ulceration

The causes and sequelae of corneal ulceration are set out below. The pathological mechanisms of the various causes of corneal ulceration are also shown in Figure 3.1.

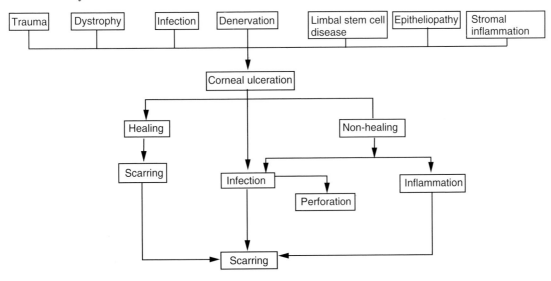

Figure 3.1   Causes and sequelae of corneal ulceration

Trauma

Trauma is the most common cause of corneal ulceration. Abrasions can result from almost any cause of injury and incisional injuries also cause epithelial loss.

Chemical injuries, ranging from minor exposure to washing up liquid to major alkali injuries, are unfortunately common. They cause ulceration by direct toxic effects on epithelial cells. Chemical burns are notoriously slow to heal.

Abrasive loss of epithelium due to blunt trauma can be extensive but tends to heal quickly unless complicated by infection or excessive topical medication.

Dystrophic changes

Dystrophic changes of various types may result in corneal ulceration. Inherited corneal dystrophies affecting the superficial cornea, such as anterior membrane dystrophy, Reis–Bückler's, lattice, macular, and granular dystrophy, can all be complicated by spontaneous corneal ulceration. So too can dystrophic epithelium present in areas of previous ulceration. Such epithelium fails to develop effective adherence to the underlying structures and is prone to recurrent ulceration.

Infection

Infection is seldom a cause of epithelial loss except with herpes simplex virus infection of the epithelium which can result in dendritic or geographic ulceration. Bacteria, fungi, and acanthamoeba all require a damaged epithelium to gain entry to the eye. The predisposing pathology may be pre-existing macroulceration, as occurs when bacterial infection complicates an abrasion, or a minor degree of epithelial abnormality, as when amoebic infection complicates contact lens wear.

Stem cell insufficiency

Limbal disease can be associated with a deficiency of epithelial stem cells, which can result in recurrent central corneal epithelial disease, including recurrent or intractable ulceration.

Epitheliopathy

Epitheliopathy, due to either environmental factors or inherently defective differentiation of limbal stem cells to terminal differentiated surface of epithelium, can result in a tendency to ulcerate. Epithelial growth and differentiation are under complex control, even under physiological conditions. Soluble factors, local matrix conditions, contact with surrounding cells and sensory innervation all affect epithelial growth and differentiation. Under pathological conditions, the normal control mechanisms are distorted. There may be direct cytopathic effects, as occur with viral infection, altered nutrition and oxygenation through tear film disturbance or recurrent trauma, as might occur with trichiasis or contact lens wear.

Denervation

Denervation has a powerful effect on the growth and differentiation of corneal epithelial nerves and anaesthetic corneas are particularly prone to recalcitrant ulceration. The precise cause of this is not known but it is assumed that neuropeptides contained in the nerves have a role in maintaining the epithelium.

Stromal inflammation

Stromal inflammation can cause and prolong corneal ulceration. Peripheral stromal cellular infiltrates are often the cause of peripheral corneal ulceration. The epithelium cannot survive over a focus of intense, superficial stromal inflammation. Similarly, stromal inflammation in herpetic keratitis may prevent the epithelium from healing; the inflamed stroma is an inappropriate support for healing epithelium. Persistent ulceration in this situation is referred to as metaherpetic ulceration.

A summary of the cellular mechanisms leading to corneal ulceration from various causes is shown in Box 3.1.

Sequelae of corneal ulceration

Healing is the most common sequel of corneal ulceration. Under uncomplicated circumstances, epithelial defects, however large, can heal within 24–48 hours. This process can be slowed by drug toxicity, infection, inflammation of the stroma, or epitheliopathy of one type or another.

Infection is the most serious complication of corneal ulceration. The corneal epithelium is an essential defence against microbial invasion and the infection which can result from inoculation of organisms, whether at the time of ulceration or later, when they may find their way through the epithelial defect. Inflammation of the stroma quickly ensues after the establishment of infection. This may be complicated by stromal lysis and perforation, chronic inflammation, if the infective organisms are of low virulence, or scarring.

Inflammation may occur without infection. Exposed stroma soon becomes oedematous and inflamed. This too may lead to scarring.

Scarring may occur after normal healing, particularly if there has been stromal injury, or after acute or chronic inflammation.

Clinical assessment of corneal ulceration

An effective clinical assessment will usually reveal the presence and cause of corneal ulceration. In most cases, a careful history will reveal the nature of the problem.

History

The key points to be identified when talking with the patient are whether there is a history of trauma or a history of recurrence which might suggest a dystrophy, recurrent erosion, or herpetic epithelial disease. Previous herpetic eye disease may point to recurrent herpetic ulceration.

Contact lens wear is also relevant. Those wearing contact lenses are prone to corneal

---

Box 3.1 *Cellular mechanisms accounting for corneal ulceration from various causes*

Epithelial cell loss	Trauma
	Chemical injury
Impaired epithelial adherence	Dystrophic condition
	Reis–Bückler dystrophy
	Granular
	Macular
	Lattice dystrophy
	Anterior membrane
	Recurrent erosion syndrome
	Diabetes
Impaired epithelial cell replacement	Limbal insufficiency
Direct cytopathic effect on epithelium	Viral diseases (HSV)
	Bacteria
	Fungi
	Amoeba
Denervation	Trigeminal nerve lesion
	Herpes zoster ophthalmicus
Disturbed epithelial nutrition	Tear film disorder
	Corneal exposure
Disrupted stromal support	Stromal inflammation

ulceration from hypoxia due to overwear, trauma due to poor lens fit, or infection.

Previous chemical injury may suggest limbal insufficiency with epitheliopathy and a history of chronic or recurrent conjunctivitis can point to conditions which compromise the corneal epithelium by one mechanism or another. Pemphigoid, Stevens–Johnson syndrome, and trachoma can be complicated by corneal ulceration.

More acute forms of conjunctivitis, for example vernal conjunctivitis, can also affect the precorneal tear film and the integrity of the corneal epithelium.

Denervation in adults results from neurological disease affecting the trigeminal nerve and its connections, neurosurgical intervention for such things as facial pain and acoustic neuromas, and previous herpes zoster ophthalmicus. In children, congenital aplasia of the trigeminal nerve is the most common cause of corneal anaesthesia which is complicated by corneal ulceration.

It is also important to establish the length of the history and the cadence of the process. Rapidly progressive ulcers are more likely to be infected. Any story of purulent discharge also suggests infection.

Examination

It is important to take a general overview of the patient before looking specifically at the cornea. Any asymmetry of face shape or movement may be relevant, as may the posture and movement of the eyelids. At the same time, one can compare the inflammatory response of the affected eye with the other eye. An inflamed eye can be seen better with the naked eye across the room than at the slit lamp.

Corneal sensation must be tested before going on to look at the cornea and before any drops are instilled. This can be done simply by assessing the corneal reflex with a wisp of cotton wool, quantifying it with an anaesthesiometer.

Slit lamp examination is necessary to determine the size and shape of the ulcer and the nature of the edge and base. Corneal ulcers may

be large or small, central or peripheral, and broad or linear in shape. They may have a normal or abnormal stromal base, with impacted mucus and debris.

Of the broad ulcers, those less than 2 mm across are considered microulcers and those greater than 2 mm across, at any point, are described as macroulcers.

Macroulceration occurs with abrasion and erosion, and with infection. Bacteria, fungi, and acanthamoeba all cause macroulceration, as can herpes simplex virus infection when it causes a geographic ulcer.

Linear ulcers can also be due to herpes simplex virus infection when it results in dendritic ulceration. Other causes of linear ulceration include a foreign body under the upper lid, the healing of a macroulcer immediately prior to epithelial closure, and, rarely, tyrosinaemia type II.

Plaques of mucus and debris may become impacted in the base of a corneal ulcer. This occurs in patients with vernal conjunctivitis who are prone to secrete excessive amounts of tenacious mucus. Such ulcers are referred to as *shield ulcers*. Mucus plaques can also occur on intact but abnormal epithelium, as in herpes zoster ophthalmicus where plaques are laid down which have a linear branching pattern with a superficial resemblance to dendritic ulceration.

Peripheral corneal ulcers may be extensive or small and multiple. Extensive peripheral interstitial keratitis can be complicated by necrosis and ulceration. More commonly, recurrent limbal inflammation, often associated with blepharoconjunctivitis, results in peripheral corneal infiltrates and subsequent ulceration. A broad classification of the various morphological types of corneal ulcer is shown in Figure 3.2.

The edge of a corneal ulcer deserves close examination as it may reveal information about the underlying process.

Healing epithelial defects have an irregular edge with fronds of healing epithelium moving in to cover the defect. The obvious punctate epithelial erosions behind the advancing edge are indicative of rapid epithelial slide (Figure 3.3).

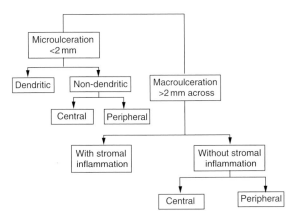

Figure 3.2 Broad classification of the morphological characteristics of common corneal ulcers

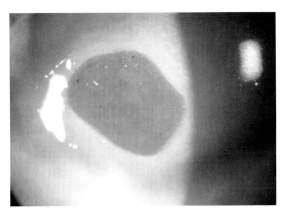

Figure 3.4 A chronic non-healing corneal ulcer with a typical rolled edge and few epithelial erosions

Chronic, non-healing ulcers tend to have a regular but elevated and rolled edge and few epithelial erosions (Figure 3.4). However, if the whole cornea is affected by drug toxicity, the whole epithelium is covered with erosions.

Objective examination of the base of the ulcer is particularly important. The base may be normal stroma, as seen with healing abrasions, there may be some oedema and chronic inflammatory changes, as seen with persistent epithelial defects which have existed for more than four or five days, or there may be acute inflammation with suppuration (Figure 3.5). Oedema and dense cellular infiltration in the base of a corneal ulcer suggest infection.

It is also important to examine the entire ocular surface remote from the corneal ulcer. Other non-ulcerated areas of the epithelium may suggest the underlying cause of the ulcer and it is, of course, mandatory to carefully examine the other eye for the same reason. Subepithelial scarring suggests a recurring process, perhaps of herpetic origin, due to recurrent erosions. Similarly, subconjunctival scarring may suggest a more widespread process leading to the corneal epithelium being compromised. The presence of trichiasis or a subtarsal foreign body is also a relevant finding, as is a history of contact lens wear.

The relationship of factors uncovered by history and examination is set out in Tables 3.1 and 3.2.

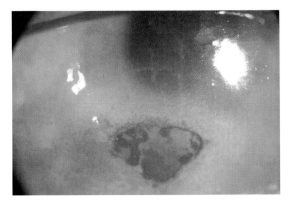

Figure 3.3 Corneal ulcer with an active and healing edge. The epithelial margin is irregular with fronds of advancing epithelium and punctate epithelial erosions behind the healing edge, suggesting epithelial sliding

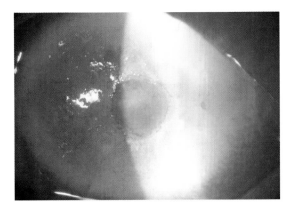

Figure 3.5 A corneal ulcer may fail to heal because of inflammation in the underlying corneal stroma

Table 3.1 Possible implications of features of history in patients with corneal ulceration

Finding	Suggests
Trauma	Abrasion
Recurrence	Dystrophy
	Recurrent erosion
	Herpetic epithelial disease
Contact lens wear	Microbial keratitis
Pervious chemical injury	Limbal insufficiency
Allergic disease	Shield ulcer
Neurological disease	Neurotrophic ulceration
Previous HZO	Neurotrophic ulceration
Discharge	Microbial keratitis
Prolonged use of eye drops	Drug toxicity
Length of history <7 days	Acute process
Length of history >7 days	More chronic process

Is the cornea infected? A diagnostic priority

The most important decision to be made based on the clinical findings is whether a corneal ulcer is infected. Corneal infection is an ophthalmic emergency which, left unrecognised and untreated, can result in blindness and loss of an eye, within hours in some cases. For this reason, microbial keratitis must be excluded as the first priority when assessing patients with ocular inflammation.

Acute stromal inflammation suggests infection. Bacteria and some fungi are potent stimulators of acute inflammation. All patients with corneal ulceration and stromal inflammation should be thought of as infected and the pathogen sought by appropriate microbiological investigations. Patients with a short history, acute inflammation of the stroma, and an anterior chamber reaction are more likely to yield organisms (Figure 3.6).

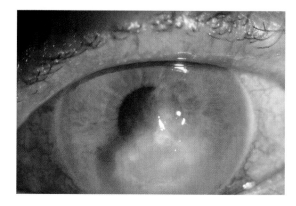

Figure 3.6 Infected corneal ulcer. There is stromal inflammation, a brisk anterior chamber reaction, and a rapidly evolving course

Table 3.2 Possible implications of clinical signs in patients with corneal ulceration

Examination	Finding	Implication
General observation	Abnormal lid position or function	Exposure
Corneal sensitivity	Decreased	Neurotrophic ulcer
Slit lamp examination		
Site	Central	All causes *except* blepharokeratoconjunctivitis
	Peripheral	Blepharokeratoconjunctivitis
		Ischaemia due to arteritis
		Mooren's
Size	>2 mm macroulcer	Abrasion, erosion, infection
	<2 mm microulcer	
Shape	Geographic	Abrasion, erosion, infection
	Linear	Herpes simplex virus
		Foreign body under lid
Edge	Irregular with "fronds" of epithelium	Healing ulcer
	Regular, rounded, elevated	Chronic ulceration
Base	Normal	Acute ulceration
	Inflamed	Infection
Anterior chamber	Inflammation ± hypopyon	Infection
Conjunctiva	Submucosal fibrosis	Chronic ocular surface condition, e.g. pemphigoid

Microbiological investigation of a suspicious corneal ulcer: some preliminary issues

Corneal scrapings are taken at the slit lamp. A drop of non-preserved local anaesthetic is instilled prior to collecting the specimens. Multiple collections are made from the edge of the ulcer and the base using a platinum spatula. One scraping is taken for each smear and each microbiological medium, flaming the spatula between each scraping (Figure 3.7).

If, on the other hand, the patient has had symptoms for more than two weeks and the cornea is inflamed, but not acutely in that there is no hypopyon and minimal oedema in the surrounding non-ulcerated cornea, other explanations may be plausible. For example, chronic herpetic keratitis or drug toxicity in someone who may well have been infected initially are alternative causes of this clinical pattern. In such cases, it is desirable to exclude infection and the only way to do this is with microbiological investigations.

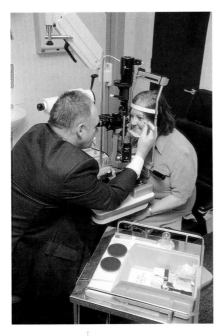

Figure 3.7 Specimen collection from a patient suspected of having an infected corneal ulcer. A "mobile" satellite laboratory facilitates the process

Two approaches are reasonable. The first is to investigate immediately, the second is to withdraw all medication, observe the patient over 24 hours and carry out the microbiological investigations, then see if the patient is worse or has failed to improve. Whether to investigate immediately or delay for 24 hours depends on the likelihood of infection being present, the anticipated morbidity from collecting the microbiological material and whether the patient has been receiving topical antibiotics. If the patient has received topical antibiotics, the chance of recovering an organism, even an organism continuing to cause disease, is very small. It is usually preferable to withhold all treatment for 24 hours before trying to recover organisms. Withdrawal of topical medication in patients with a longer (greater than two weeks) history often results in a marked improvement because the major influence on the chronic inflammation and poor epithelial healing is drug toxicity. If the patient is no worse after withdrawal of topical medication for 24 hours, it is safe to withhold medication for a further period until the problem has either resolved or progressed. If the pathology has progressed, a corneal biopsy is indicated. This approach is summarised in Figure 3.8. Microbial keratitis is considered in detail on p. 55.

Having excluded infection in patients with an inflamed eye and corneal ulceration, the other patterns of corneal ulceration can be considered.

Non-microbial ulcerative keratitis

Infection is unlikely if there is corneal ulceration but no stromal inflammation. Similarly, in cases where there is ulceration and chronic inflammation, factors other than infection may be operating.

Acute corneal ulceration with uninflamed stroma may be due to trauma, recurrent spontaneous erosion, or cytopathic changes in the epithelium caused by herpes simplex virus. These conditions can usually be differentiated by the history or, in the case of herpes simplex

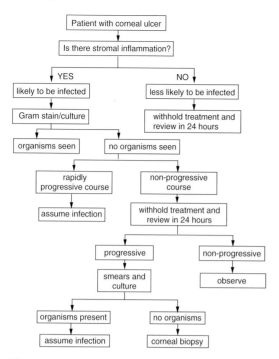

Figure 3.8 Strategy for deciding whether a corneal ulcer is infected

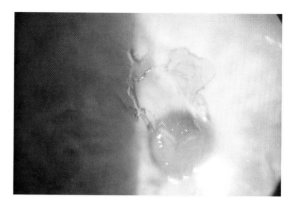

Figure 3.9 Recurrent erosion complicating previous trauma

infection, there may be a characteristic dendritic ulcer.

Chronic corneal ulceration may result from impaired corneal healing as a consequence of limbal stem cell deficiency, denervation or drug toxicity. Dystrophic conditions and repeated ulceration may damage the adhesive mechanisms of epithelial cells and discourage healing.

Recurrent erosion syndrome

Recurrent spontaneous ulceration of the cornea may result from trauma, especially injuries from fingernails, paper, or twigs. It may also result from dystrophies, particularly anterior membrane dystrophy, Reis–Bückler's, and stromal dystrophies such as lattice, granular and, less commonly, macular dystrophy.

Epithelial instability can also result from chemical or thermal injury, previous infection, such as herpetic keratitis, degenerations, such as Saltzmann's degeneration and band keratopathy, and a number of other processes, such as keratoconjunctivitis sicca, exposure, neurotrophic keratitis, and bullous keratopathy. Diabetics are also prone to spontaneous corneal ulceration.

Usually patients with recurrent erosion syndrome experience pain on awakening in the morning. The disease occurs in two forms. In the minor form, there are microcystic changes or perhaps small detachments which may prove impossible to see. In these cases, symptoms usually resolve in a few hours. In the more severe form, there is frank ulceration which may be extensive. This major form tends to complicate previous trauma (Figure 3.9).

Management involves determining the cause and treating any underlying condition as required. It also involves providing maintenance treatment between attacks. This includes the use of ocular lubricants at night and, in some cases, the use of soft, thin, high-water content contact lenses as a splinting bandage.

Surgical intervention may be indicated to remove loose epithelium or create epithelial–stromal adhesions by micropuncture. Both of these procedures can be done at the slit lamp. The simplest way to perform micropuncture is with a 23 gauge needle. Multiple punctures made in the area of epithelial instability are best done between erosive episodes.

Dendritic ulceration

Herpes simplex virus infection is the usual cause of dendritic ulceration of the cornea. The branching linear defects in the epithelium are the result of the direct cytopathic effect of the virus on the corneal epithelium. Epithelial cells removed from the edge of the ulcer and examined by electron microscopy are seen to be laden with viral particles. As the infected cells die, virus particles infect adjacent cells to produce a linear pattern of epitheliopathy. Infected cells may be shed to the extent that Bowman's membrane is exposed, creating a true dendritic ulcer. Quite often, the infected epithelial cells are not shed but the cytopathic effect of the virus on the cells is readily seen in a dendritic pattern. These lesions are also referred to as dendritic ulcers, but this is incorrect in the strict sense of the word (Figure 3.10).

Dendritic ulcers due to herpes simplex virus may be large or small, single or multiple. Micro-dendrites (less than 0.5 mm in length) tend to be multiple. Usually the stroma beneath the ulcer is not inflamed but inflammation may occur in recurrent cases or with immunocompromised patients. Herpetic disease is usually unilateral but it may be bilateral in the immunocompromised, particularly in atopic patients.

Atopic individuals have deficient mucosal surface immunity and are prone to severe herpetic corneal disease. So too are those who have their ocular surface immunity impaired by the use of topical corticosteroids. In this group of patients, the virus moves from one cell to another very easily, causing widespread corneal

epithelial loss and resulting in a geographic ulcer. In addition, the stroma is more frequently involved (Figure 3.11).

Entities other than herpes simplex virus which cause dendritic epithelial lesions are healing epithelial defects, varicella-zoster infection, and tyrosinaemia type II. Healing defects create dendritic lesions at the point of epithelial closure. A history of corneal ulceration and careful examination of the advancing epithelial edge will distinguish this lesion from dendritic ulceration due to herpes simplex infection (Figures 3.12 and 3.13).

Tyrosinaemia type II also causes dendritic lesions in the corneal epithelium but not with ulceration. In these cases, the epitheliopathy is due to metabolic products and is bilateral, although not necessarily dendritic on both sides. The patients usually have mild mental retardation and hyperkeratosis in the palms of the hands and the soles of the feet (Figure 3.14).

Varicella-zoster dendritic keratopathy is usually due to mucus plaques forming on abnormal epithelium (Figure 3.15). The concurrent use of rose bengal 1% solution eye drops and fluorescein eye drops will identify these lesions because they have a characteristic appearance. The linear branching mucus plaque stains intensely with the rose bengal and the fluorescein pools around the edges. This is the

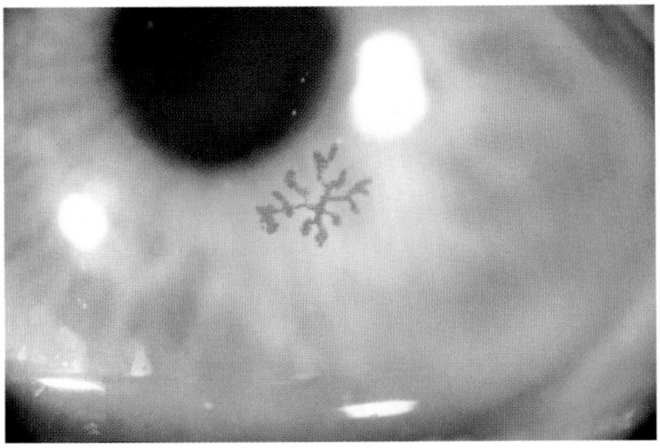

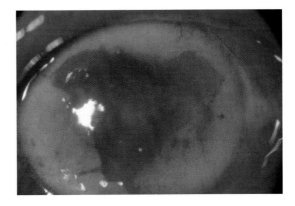

Figure 3.10 A dendritic figure created by the cytopathic effect of herpes simplex virus on corneal epithelial cells. In this case cells have not been shed to create an ulcer

Figure 3.11 Geographic ulcer due to herpes simplex virus infection. The transmission of virus to adjacent cells has created a large area of severe cytopathic effect with extensive cell loss and geographic ulceration

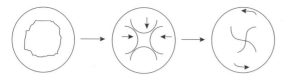

Figure 3.12 A healing epithelial defect may produce a dendritic figure. Epithelial cells move from the edge of the epithelial defect centrally and tangentially. As the edges meet a dendritic figure may be produced

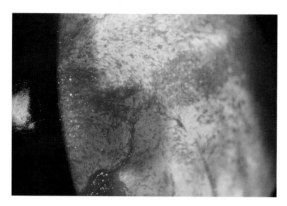

Figure 3.13 A branching linear figure with surrounding vortex pattern created by a healing epithelial defect

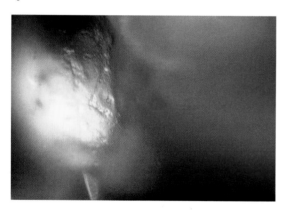

Figure 3.14 Dendritic keratopathy in a patient with tyrosinaemia type II

reverse of what is found with a true dendritic ulcer, where the base stains with fluorescein and the edge with rose bengal (Figure 3.16).

Geographic ulceration

Macroulceration can occur as a consequence of herpes simplex virus infection when conditions favour the virus for the reasons mentioned above. For purposes of classification,

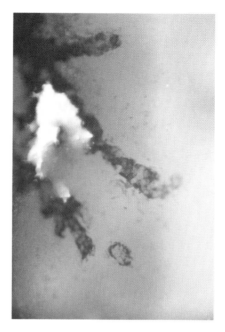

Figure 3.15 Dendritic mucus plaque in a patient with herpes zoster ophthalmicus

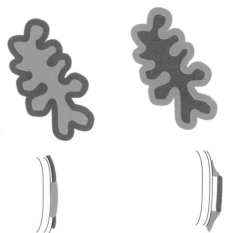

Herpes simplex keratitis   Herpes zoster ophthalmicus
Dendric keratitis   Dendriform plaque

Figure 3.16 The staining patterns with fluorescein and rose bengal differentiate the dendritic lesions of herpes simplex virus infection and herpes zoster ophthalmicus

the term "geographic" is used to describe ulcers which have a breadth of 0.5 mm at any point.

Chronic epithelial defects

There are other causes of chronic (>14 days) corneal ulceration. These include drug toxicity, limbal stem cell insufficiency, inflammation of the underlying stroma, tear film deficiency, infection with organisms of low virulence, and recurrent erosions.

The most common cause of delayed epithelial healing, and the most treatable, is drug toxicity. Patients with corneal ulceration are often over-treated with topical medication, either because the cause of the ulceration is unknown and all conceivable possibilities, such as microbial keratitis, are treated with intensive polypharmacy or treatment is prolonged beyond the point at which the organisms are eradicated.

Epithelial closure is an urgent and important milestone in the treatment of all forms of corneal ulceration, including microbial keratitis. As soon as the threat of infection is overcome, topical antibiotics should be withdrawn to encourage epithelial healing. Seldom is it necessary to continue antibiotics for more than seven days when treating bacterial keratitis. Some more fastidious bacteria, like those causing infectious crystalline keratopathy, fungi, and acanthamoeba require more prolonged therapy.

Withdrawal of topical medication is enough to encourage epithelial healing in many cases of chronic corneal ulceration.

If healing has not occurred, or is not occurring after 7–10 days, the state of the underlying stroma should be addressed. Stromal inflammation impairs epithelial wound healing. It may also indicate residual infection with a low virulence organism. Patients with stromal inflammation continuing after 10 days off all topical medication should be reinvestigated with corneal scraping and corneal biopsy, looking in particular for low virulence organisms.

If no organisms are found or if there is no stromal inflammation under the epithelial defect, the next step is to trial a soft, thin, high-water content contact lens. In some patients this will be enough to protect the epithelium from adverse external influences such as eyelid movement and to encourage epithelial healing.

Epithelial defects persisting after a trial of contact lens splinting can be given a trial of ptosis.

Botulinum injection will induce a temporary ptosis which is sometimes enough to provide protection for the epithelium and promote epithelial closure. Should all these measures fail, a conjunctival flap may prove necessary. Permanent non-healing epithelial defects are incompatible with the long term survival of the eye, so epithelial closure must somehow be achieved. A summary of measures to heal a chronic epithelial defect is set out in Figure 3.17. If medical measures fail, surgery is mandatory.

Conjunctival flaps can be complete, as described by Gunderson, where the superior bulbar conjunctiva is mobilised to cover the entire cornea, or they can be smaller, pedicled flaps that are based on the insertion of one of the recti (the

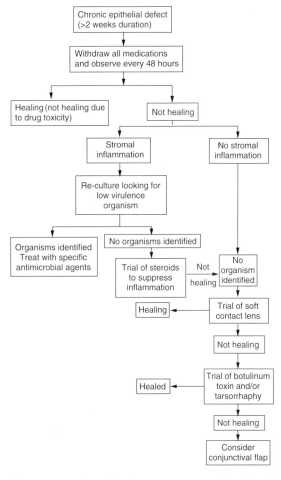

Figure 3.17 Steps in the management of a chronic epithelial defect

source of the conjunctival arterial circulation) and swung around to cover the epithelial defect.

In recent times, some new developments have been proposed for the treatment of persistent epithelial defects. These include the use of amniotic membrane grafts, limbal autografts and allografts, topical fibronectin, and autologous serum. Each of these approaches is experimental and their effectiveness requires verification.

Peripheral corneal ulceration

Peripheral ulceration of the cornea occurs in a number of distinct patterns with different and identifiable causes and occurs with sufficient frequency to be considered as a distinct pattern of corneal ulceration. Peripheral corneal ulceration may be minor, even trivial, or so severe as to cause destruction of the eye and blindness. Usually the underlying cause can be established from the clinical picture.

There are three questions which must be resolved when assessing someone with marginal corneal ulceration.

- Is there any other inflammatory activity in the affected eye?
- Is the disease mild and non-destructive or severe and threatening?
- If severe and threatening, is it part of a systemic disorder?

An algorithm for evaluating patients with peripheral corneal ulceration is set out in Figure 3.18.

Peripheral corneal ulceration with coexisting ocular inflammation

The peripheral cornea is vulnerable to inflammatory processes occurring elsewhere in the eye, particularly in the conjunctiva, lid margin, sclera, and corneal stroma. Because vascular loops from the limbal circulation are present in the peripheral stroma and submucosa, leucocytes may aggregate in the peripheral cornea when there is inflammation in the region. The leucocyte aggregation may be sufficient to be considered an abscess (euphemistically referred to in the clinical

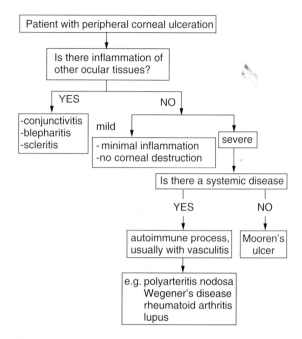

Figure 3.18 Strategy for evaluating patients with peripheral corneal ulceration

setting as an "infiltrate") around which there is inevitably oedema. These inflammatory changes in the peripheral corneal stroma affect the overlying epithelium because it requires a normal stroma for support. When the epithelium over the peripheral cornea infiltrates is lost, a peripheral corneal ulcer forms. Conjunctivitis, blepharitis, scleritis, and stromal keratitis are all associated with marginal corneal ulceration.

Blepharitis is commonly associated with peripheral corneal infiltrates and ulceration. It is proposed that blepharitis affects the corneal tear film, which in turn affects the corneal epithelium. The epithelium then loses its effectiveness as a barrier, encouraging stromal inflammation. Leucocytes are recruited through the limbal vessels and aggregate at the vascular loops in the peripheral cornea (Figure 3.19). If this inflammatory change is marked, the overlying epithelium is lost, creating a peripheral corneal ulceration.

The management of this common problem is to treat the underlying inflammatory disorder. This entails decreasing leucocyte recruitment into the limbal region by the use of topical

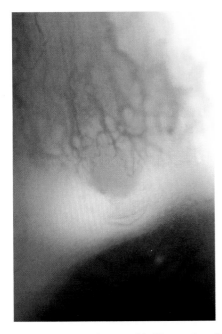

Figure 3.19 Peripheral corneal infiltrate. A collection of inflammatory cells emerging from limbal vascular loops. The overlying epithelium may break down over an infiltrate, creating a peripheral corneal ulcer

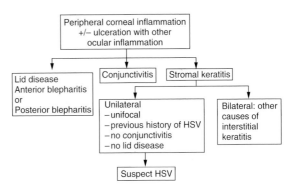

Figure 3.20 The causes of peripheral corneal inflammation and ulceration in patients with coexisting inflammatory conditions of the eye

corticosteroids. A danger entailed in this approach is the possibility of overlooking herpes simplex virus as a cause of stromal keratitis causing peripheral corneal infiltrates and ulceration. If such patients with unsuspected herpetic eye disease are given topical steroids to decrease leucocyte recruitment, there is a risk of provoking severe epithelial disease. Clinicians should be suspicious of this entity if the inflammation is confined to one eye, restricted to one locality in the affected limbus, and has occurred in the absence of inflammation of the conjunctiva and eyelids. The causes of peripheral corneal inflammation and ulceration in association with other inflammatory conditions of the eye are set out in Figure 3.20.

Peripheral corneal ulceration and inflammation without coexisting ocular inflammation

The pattern described can occur in the absence of coexisting ocular inflammation. Perhaps the pathological processes described are operating at a subclinical level or there may be other unrecognised mechanisms which await identification. In such cases, the only treatment available is a trial of topical corticosteroids using the same precautions as described in the previous section.

Peripheral corneal ulceration with severe inflammation and destruction

When limbal inflammation is severe and destructive, a search for an associated systemic disease is mandatory. Because the peripheral cornea is dependent on the limbal circulation for its integrity, diseases with an arteritic component are particularly threatening to the cornea. Rheumatoid arthritis, Wegener's granulomatosis, polyarteritis nodosa, systemic lupus erythematosus, relapsing polychondritis, giant cell arteritis, progressive systemic sclerosis, and herpes zoster ophthalmicus can all cause peripheral corneal destruction through vasculitis (Figure 3.21). Other conditions associated with the process include hepatitis C virus infection, mid-line lethal granuloma, and some blood dysplasias.

The clinical features of this type of pathology are striking. The resulting process is usually extensive, extending circumferentially to include most of the peripheral cornea, although the degree of involvement may be quite uneven. The process may also extend into the central cornea or out into

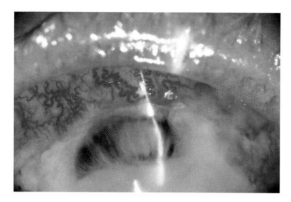

Figure 3.21 Peripheral corneal inflammation, ulceration, and corneal destruction in a patient with Wegener's granulomatosis

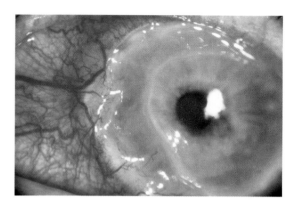

Figure 3.22 Mooren's ulcer. Peripheral corneal ulceration, inflammation, and corneal destruction in a patient in whom no systemic process can be identified. The dense aggregation of inflammatory cells in the stroma brings about the corneal destruction

the adjacent sclera. It may be unilateral or bilateral and, if the latter, can be quite asymmetrical.

To identify the underlying cause, patients with this pattern of corneal disease should be investigated thoroughly. They should have a chest radiograph, full blood examination, urea and electrolytes, rheumatoid factor, antinuclear factor, antibody to neutrophil cytoplasmic antigen (ANCA), and serology for hepatitis C virus. Careful evaluation by a physician experienced with the associated disorders, their investigation, and treatment is sometimes desirable.

Mooren's ulceration

This term is reserved for cases in which there is substantial inflammation, tissue destruction, and peripheral corneal ulceration without coexisting inflammation in the eye and with no evidence of a systemic disorder (Figure 3.22). The underlying pathological mechanism is unknown, although various immunological mechanisms have been proposed.

The management of this disorder and of similar disorders where an underlying cause has been identified is similar. Any underlying disorder must be appropriately managed and is usually achieved in cooperation with a physician. The ocular therapy involves limiting further leucocyte recruitment by the use of topical steroids, ensuring that the excavated or elevated areas of the peripheral cornea are well lubricated with tear film supplements and treating any threatening areas of tissue loss.

If perforation occurs, glue and a contact lens is the preferred option. This is usually effective for small perforations of less than 1 mm. For larger perforations, surgical repair is best achieved with a pedicled conjunctival flap. If this is not possible, repair with an autograft (periosteum or even skin) is usually better than an allograft. The problem with all free grafts, autografts or allografts is poor healing due to avascularity in the perforated area. In those having extensive, threatening disease but with no detectable underlying condition (Mooren's ulceration) it may be necessary to use systemic immunosuppression to control the disease. The choice of agents is arbitrary in that no one approach to immunosuppression has proven to be superior. Systemic steroids are often necessary but since long term therapy is frequently required, it is wise to use cyclosporin alone or in combination with other agents. This minimises the dose, and therefore the side effects, of systemic corticosteroids.

Microbial keratitis

The most important cause of corneal ulceration is microbial infection. It is important because it is threatening. As mentioned previously, whenever there is corneal ulceration and stromal inflammation, infection should be assumed until disproved by negative microbiological investigations and a resolving clinical course.

Pathogenesis

Almost invariably, microbial keratitis occurs in compromised corneas. The most common predisposing factors are trauma, bullous keratopathy, existing corneal ulceration, herpetic eye disease, severe tear film deficiency, and contact lens wear.

The common pathogens are as follows.

- Bacteria
    Staphylococcus aureus
    Staphylococcus epidermidis
    Streptococcus pneumoniae
    Streptococcus pyogenes
    Viridans streptococci
    Corynebacterium species
    Pseudomonas aeruginosa
    Moraxella species
    Haemophilus influenzae
    Proteus mirabilis
    Serratia marescens

- Fungi
    Fusarium solani
    Aspergillus species
    Acremonium species
    Alternaria species
    Penicillium species
    Candida albicans

- Protozoa
    Acanthamoeba

These organisms may derive from the commensal flora of the external eye. One or more components of the flora may take advantage of a situation to penetrate the cornea (an endogenous source of infection). Alternatively, organisms may be inoculated from the external environment at the time of injury (an exogenous source of infection).

For infection to occur, organisms must attach to the epithelium, penetrate into the stroma, replicate, and produce toxins which damage the corneal structure and initiate the host response (Figure 3.23). The host response has specific and non-specific elements. The most obvious

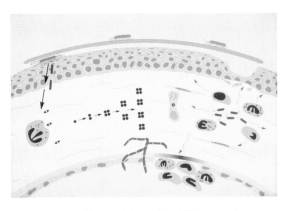

Figure 3.23 Corneal infection. The organism must attach to and penetrate the corneal surface, evade the host response, multiply, and damage the cornea directly or through toxin release. The host response also contributes to the pathology

response is recruitment of leucocytes into the infected region. This accumulation can be seen clinically and in more severe forms is described as suppuration or abscess formation. Both the organisms and the host response contribute to corneal damage, including ulceration. The clinical picture is therefore determined by the predisposing disease in the external eye, the pathogenic mechanisms of the infecting organism and the host response (Figure 3.24). In the common and fully expressed form, there is ulceration and suppuration with focal or diffuse stromal inflammation and iritis.

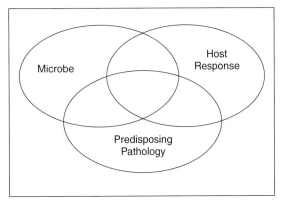

Figure 3.24 The underlying or predisposing condition, the causative organism, and the host response to infection contribute to the clinical features of microbial keratitis

Management of microbial keratitis

The key to effective management of microbial keratitis is to see the patient as early as possible in the course of the disease, to promptly identify the causative organism, and to deliver specific antimicrobial chemotherapy.

Early presentation requires that people at risk, such as those injured, contact lens wearers, and patients with corneal grafts, have easy access to specialist care. When patients present with what may be corneal infection, they must be seen promptly and the relevant investigations performed immediately. Initial therapy should be based on the clinical picture and the Gram stain.

Investigation of patients with suspected microbial keratitis

All that can be deduced from the clinical examination is whether the patient is likely to be infected or not. The aetiological agent can only be identified by the appropriate microbiological investigations. Since microbial keratitis is a threatening condition, a conservative approach is required. Any possibility of infection demands microbiological investigation. Of course, some indication of the causative organism can be gleaned from the cadence of the clinical progression. Severe destructive disease is more likely to be due to *Staphylococcus aureus*, *Streptococcus pneumoniae*, *Pseudomonas aeruginosa* and, in tropical areas, *Fusarium solani*. More slowly progressive, non-destructive disease is more likely to be due to less virulent organisms such as the following.

- Bacteria   Coagulase-negative staphylococci
  Viridans streptococci
  Corynebacteria
  Enterobacteriaceae
  Acinetobacter

- Fungi   Paecilomyces
  Penicillium
  Candida species other than
  C. albicans

Because the clinical features are not usually characteristic of a particular organism, it is preferable to ignore them for the purpose of selecting the initial therapy. The selection of initial therapy is based on the Gram stain and the clinical features. The underlying assumption must be that the cornea is infected with the most threatening organism. The Gram stain is therefore a critical step in the selection of the initial therapy.

Collection of material for microbiological assessment

Material is collected from the cornea as soon as infection is suspected. To encourage this and to ensure specimens collected are managed optimally, a satellite laboratory should be established in the clinic where patients with corneal infections present. All that is required for collecting specimens should be assembled on a trolley and wheeled to the side of the slit lamp at which the examination is to be conducted (Figure 3.25). If the microbiological media are kept in a refrigerator, it is best to allow them to warm to room temperature before inoculation. A standard plan for collection of specimens should be employed for all patients.

A drop of non-preserved local anaesthetic is instilled prior to collecting the specimens of corneal scrapings at the slit lamp. Multiple collections are made from the edge of the ulcer and from the base using a platinum spatula.

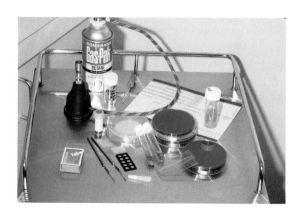

Figure 3.25 Equipment required for specimen collection

Ideally, one scraping is taken for each microbiological medium, flaming the spatula and allowing about 20 seconds for the tip to cool between each scraping. If a platinum spatula is not available, another flexible instrument such as a hypodermic needle can be used, but this is not as effective.

Material collected is distributed into media as follows.

- Chocolate agar   Incubated in air 15% CO_2 at 35°C
- Blood agar   Incubated an-aerobically at 35°C
- Gram stain   –
- Sabouraud's agar   Incubated in air at 28°C
- Special brain-heart infusion broth   Incubated in air 15% CO_2 at 35°C
- Cooked meat medium   Incubated an-aerobically at 35°C

If further scrapings are possible, a second slide for a Giemsa stain may be prepared and a second plate for blood agar. The clinician may choose to use the "C streak" method of inoculating agar plates or to spread material on one side of a plate and allow streaking out to be done in the laboratory. The Sabouraud agar is best inoculated by making several shallow stabs. The broths are inoculated by twirling the spatula vigorously, being careful to avoid contamination by the handle of the instrument. The smears are air dried and then fixed; Gram stains are usually heat fixed and Giemsa stains methanol fixed. This is best done in the laboratory but, if necessary, the clinician may heat-fix a smear by quickly passing the slide twice through a flame. Do not attempt to heat-fix a wet smear. Mark the slide so that it is clear which side is "up". Inoculated media should be transported to the laboratory without delay, especially if anaerobes are suspected.

The Gram stain

The Gram stain is usually done in the laboratory, but it is sometimes necessary for the ophthalmologist to stain the specimen and examine it; the method is set out in Chapter 14.

If organisms are seen in the Gram stain, the cornea should be considered infected until proven otherwise. If the Gram stain is negative but the clinical features suggest infection, the same assumption should be made. Looking at Gram stains from corneal infections requires experience; the presence of one or two organisms is enough to confirm a clinical suspicion of infection. In general microbiology, infection usually results in many more organisms being seen, for example, in pus or urine specimens. Gram stains from corneal infections should be examined by someone experienced with eye specimens; that is, either a microbiologist or an ophthalmologist familiar with the process. Initial therapy is based on the Gram stain result.

The Gram stain may yield a number of possible results. There may or may not be organisms. If there are organisms, the cornea is almost always infected. If there are no organisms, the cornea may still be infected. If the clinical picture suggests that this is likely, the negative Gram stain should be ignored and infection assumed.

The issue to be resolved from the Gram stain is whether organisms are present and, if so, whether they are bacteria, fungi, or acanthamoeba.

Bacterial infection is much more common than fungal or amoebic infection. If bacteria are present in the smear, all that can be reliably ascertained is whether they are Gram positive or Gram negative and whether they are cocci or rods. Although some organisms have characteristic appearances in stains, it is safer not to attempt to specifically identify bacteria from smears but merely to ascertain their Gram staining characteristics and whether fungi are yeasts or filamentous forms.

Initial therapy is based on the Gram stain, assuming the worst possibility. If there are Gram positive cocci in the smear, it is assumed that the cornea is infected with a *Staphylococcus aureus* producing penicillinase and it is treated accordingly (Figure 3.26). If there are Gram negative bacilli in the smear, it is assumed that

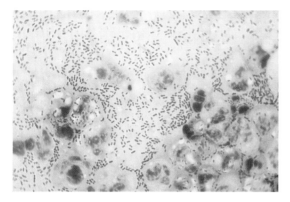

Figure 3.26   Gram stain with large numbers of Gram positive cocci. A more specific microbial diagnosis cannot be made from the Gram stain

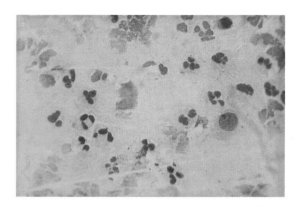

Figure 3.28   Gram stain. No definite organisms can be seen

the cornea is infected with *Pseudomonas aeruginosa* (Figure 3.27). If the clinical picture is of infection but organisms are not seen in the smear (Figure 3.28), it is assumed that there is a mixed infection, including the worst two possibilities: *Staphylococcus aureus* producing penicillinase and *Pseudomonas aeruginosa*.

Figure 3.27   Gram stain with large numbers of Gram negative bacilli. A more specific microbiological diagnosis cannot be made from the Gram stain

Culture results

With the initial therapy based on the Gram stain, it is necessary to consider modifying therapy when the culture results become available in 24 hours and perhaps to modify therapy further when antibiotic sensitivities become clear in another 24 hours. Any requirement to alter the initial antimicrobial chemotherapy should be based on the clinical course. If the course is favourable, nothing needs to be changed. If not, and the organism isolated might be more sensitive to another agent or if the pattern of antibiotic sensitivity suggests another agent, changes to the initial therapy should be made.

Antibiotic sensitivity data for organisms causing bacterial keratitis need cautious assessment. The level of antibiotic achievable in the infected cornea using topical application is much higher than can safely be achieved in blood from parenteral administration. The choice of antibiotics for treating microbial keratitis is set out in Table 3.3.

Corneal biopsy in ulcerative keratitis

Repeated failed attempts to isolate pathogens from patients with persistent ulceration and chronic inflammation suggest that offending organisms are deep in the cornea and not accessible to scrapings. For these patients corneal biopsy is necessary.

Table 3.3 Antibacterial preparations used to treat bacterial keratitis

	Commercial preparation	Fortified
Cephalothin	–	50 mg/ml
Gentamicin	3 mg/ml	15 mg/ml
Ciprofloxacin	3 mg/ml	
Ofloxacin	3 mg/ml	
Penicillin G		5000 U/ml(0.3%)
Tobramycin	3 mg/ml	15 mg/ml
Vancomycin		50 mg/ml

Corneal biopsy can be done in several ways. It can be done at the slit lamp using an unpreserved topical anaesthetic agent; a small 2–3 mm trephine is used to incise approximately 30% corneal depth and the central stump is amputated with a diamond knife. Alternatively, the procedure can be done under an operating microscope; instead of trephining, the desired area can be cut out using a diamond knife. The specimen is then divided into three portions: one for microbiology, one for light microscopy, and the third for electron microscopy (Figure 3.29).

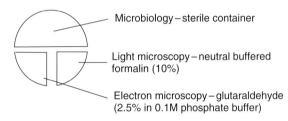

Microbiology – sterile container

Light microscopy – neutral buffered formalin (10%)

Electron microscopy – glutaraldehyde (2.5% in 0.1M phosphate buffer)

Figure 3.29 Management of a corneal biopsy done to investigate infection. Half the specimen is put into a sterile container and sent to the forewarned microbiologist. The other half is processed for light and electron microscopy

Selection of antimicrobial chemotherapy

The selection of an antibiotic for a patient considered to be infected is based on the clinical picture: whether the cornea is likely to be infected, the Gram stain, and the preference and protocols of the ophthalmologist. A number of selections are possible but the choice usually comes down to a combination of a topical aminoglycoside (e.g. gentamicin 14 mg/ml) and a second generation cephalosporin (e.g. cephalothin 50 mg/ml) or monotherapy with a fluoroquinalone (e.g. ciprofloxacin or ofloxacin).

Although the combination of aminoglycoside and cephalosporin has slightly broader bacterial susceptibility than fluoroquinolones, the latter are not so effective against streptococci, but are more convenient to use. The combined medication, which is more effective in fortified concentrations, must be made up individually for each patient because the cephalosporins are unstable and must be made up afresh every 4–5 days. Despite this inconvenience, many prefer to use the combination therapy rather than monotherapy because of its broad coverage which is advantageous in the initial phase of treatment.

If the Gram stain provides an unequivocal result, one element of the combination therapy may be omitted from the outset. For example, if there are only Gram negative bacilli in the smear, the cephalosporin need not be given.

The second opportunity to modify the selection of antibiotic comes with the result of culture, which is generally available 24 hours after innoculation. At this stage, similar judgements can be made to those described above.

A third opportunity to modify treatment comes when the antibiotic sensitivity of the organism is identified, usually 48 hours after the scrapings were innoculated, but it is very unusual to modify therapy at this stage. The initial selection is usually effective and even unexpectedly resistant strains are susceptible at the very high tissue levels achieved with intensive topical medication.

Initially, topical antibiotics should be given every hour for the first 24 hours, then hourly during the day for the next three days. Given a satisfactory clinical response, the frequency of administration can be reduced to four times a day after the fourth day and ceased at the seventh day. Patients should be seen daily for the first two days and again on the seventh day when the cessation of the antibiotics is planned. Patients should also be seen 24 hours after this to ensure that the withdrawal of medication has not been complicated by recurrence.

There is no point in resorting to subconjunctival injections or systemic therapy. However, systemic therapy should be considered if the sclera is involved in the infective process.

The place of topical corticosteroids in the treatment of microbial keratitis

The place of topical corticosteroids in the treatment of bacterial keratitis remains controversial. Much of the damage to the cornea in cases of microbial keratitis results from the host response. Leucocytes are recruited to the site of infection and release lytic enzymes into the stroma. Although this recruitment can be limited by the use of topical corticosteroids, neutrophils in particular are essential for eradication of organisms. Furthermore, the recruitment of leucocytes due to microbial influences is often complete by the time the patient has presented and antimicrobial chemotherapy has commenced. Hence, there may be little to gain from the use of corticosteroids in addition to antibiotics. There is little evidence from clinical studies to suggest whether or not corticosteroids are useful.

There are some laboratory data which should be considered. *In vivo* experiments reveal that corticosteroids reduce the number of leucocytes recruited into the infected cornea and that the effect is greater if they are given early in the course of the infection. Furthermore, corticosteroids do not compromise the ability of an appropriate antibiotic to reduce the number of organisms in an infected cornea. However, if steroids are used in a cornea infected with Pseudomonas that is not receiving antibiotics, the infective process is accentuated; the number of bacteria in the cornea is far greater than in corneas not receiving corticosteroids. The same experiment done on animals infected with *Staphylococcus aureus* showed no compromise as a consequence of steroid administration. Whether the reduction of leucocyte recruitment achievable with corticosteroids has any long term structural consequences remains undetermined.

Based on these findings, it is reasonable to manage patients with bacterial keratitis with topical antibiotics alone. It is also reasonable to use corticosteroids to reduce the leucocyte recruitment occurring later in the natural history of the disease. At this time, the stimulus for recruitment is tissue breakdown rather than the response to bacterial replication occurring early in the disease.

Corticosteroids (topical prednisolone phosphate 0.5% four times a day) may be used, commencing once the organism has been identified and the patient has shown a satisfactory response to the initial antibiotic treatment. This usually means beginning topical corticosteroids on the second day after presentation and their cessation when antibiotics are withdrawn seven days later.

Specific forms of microbial keratitis

Infectious crystalline keratopathy

Infection of the cornea with organisms considered to be of very low virulence can occur under favourable circumstances. For example, patients who have had a corneal graft have a portal of entry (the suture track), a retained foreign body (the suture), are receiving topical immunosuppression (corticosteroids) which limits leucocyte recruitment and are sometimes receiving antibiotics, which select resistant organisms in the commensal population (Figure 3.30).

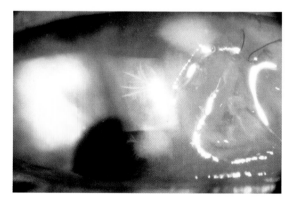

Figure 3.30 Infectious crystalline keratopathy in a patient who has had lamellar corneal transplantation for corneoscleral necrosis

Infectious crystalline keratopathy occurs in this and similar situations. Mildly pathogenic organisms invade the cornea and replicate, but attract little if any host response. They are unaffected by most antibiotic therapies. Colonies of bacteria grow into the cornea, usually through interlamellar spaces, and can be seen as linear, crystal-like structures in the stroma (Figure 3.31). The condition can resemble low grade fungal infection.

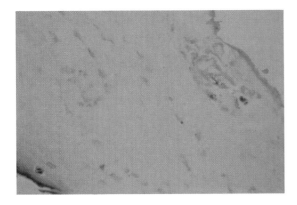

Figure 3.31 Histological section of cornea in a patient who developed infectious crystalline keratopathy after lamellar transplantation. The aggregations of bacteria have little inflammatory reaction around them

Diagnosis demands isolation of the aetiological agent. Many different organisms have been identified as causing the condition, but most commonly they are encapsulated streptococci. Scrapings should be taken for microscopy and culture and processed in the usual way. The laboratory should be made aware that an Abiotrophia species (formerly nutrient variant streptococci) may be the aetiological agent and that the cultures may therefore need extended culture or vitamin B_6 supplementation.

Treatment depends on the causative organism. An appropriate antibiotic needs to be given for a prolonged period in most cases. Because the organisms responsible for the pathology turn over slowly, prolonged therapy is usually necessary. A dosage schedule that can be tolerated in the long term is required. For example, when treating nutrient variant streptococci, penicillin (5000 U/ml) drops four times a day are effective.

Fungal keratitis

Fungal keratitis is less common than bacterial keratitis, but it is relatively more common in tropical regions and in patients with chronic corneal disorders and immunosuppression. A wide range of fungi have been implicated in corneal infections (Figures 3.32 and 3.33).

The clinical features of fungal keratitis are similar to bacterial keratitis, including macroulceration, stromal inflammation, often with suppuration, and anterior chamber inflammation, but the rate of progress is slower. Occasionally bundles of hyphae can be observed in the stroma, the appearance being similar to that seen with infectious crystalline keratopathy (Figures 3.32 and 3.33).

Because antifungal therapy is relatively non-specific, with high toxicity and relatively low killing rates for many fungi, treatment should not be instituted until a fungus is seen in the smear or isolated.

If a fungus is suspected, one smear should be stained by the Giemsa method. In communities where fungal keratitis occurs, Giemsa or acridine orange stains should be used together with the Gram stain in all cases.

Treatment of fungal keratitis is complicated because the susceptibility of the different

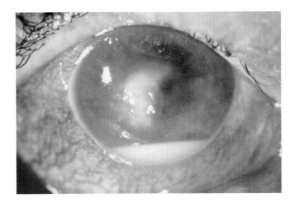

Figure 3.32 Fungal keratitis. Corneal infection with *Fusarium solani*

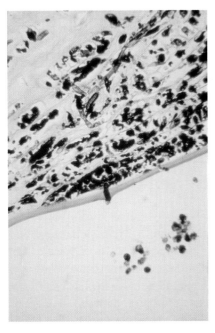

Figure 3.33 Fungal keratitis. Histological section of cornea stained with silver to demonstrate filamentous forms

Table 3.4 Antifungal agents used to treat fungal keratitis

Microscopic features	Examples	Drug choice
Filamentous	Aspergillus	Natamycin 5% drops
	Fusarium	Miconazole 1% drops
	Penicillium	
	Culveria	
	Acremonium	Consider oral ketaconazole 400 mg/day
	Paecilomyces	
	Cladosporium	
Yeast	Candida spp	Flucytosine 1% drops Miconazole 1% drops Oral flucytosine 100 mg/kg/day

fungi to the limited range of antifungal agents is unpredictable compared to bacteria and because the agents that are available are relatively toxic (Table 3.4).

Typically, topical agents are used hourly for 3–4 days until there is a clinical response and then four times a day for weeks or even months.

Sometimes it is feasible to resect the area of cornea affected, thereby reducing the mass of infection and increasing the effectiveness of antifungal chemotherapy.

When the infection is not controlled and perforation threatens, corneal transplantation may be possible and debridement and repair with a conjunctival flap is an option. Although a case can be made for the use of topical corticosteroids in the treatment of bacterial keratitis, this is not the case with fungal keratitis. Topical corticosteroids are contraindicated in fungal keratitis.

Acanthamoeba keratitis

In nature, acanthamoeba exist in two forms: either as trophozoites, which are uninucleate motile organisms about 20 mm in diameter, or as smaller double walled cysts. In adverse conditions, the trophozoites encyst and re-emerge when conditions are favourable.

Although relatively common today, acanthamoeba keratitis was not recognised until 1973. Infection with acanthamoeba causes a chronic macroulcerative keratitis with stromal inflammation.

There is often a history of contact lens wear and infection follows contamination of the lens care regimen, a particular hazard being home made saline solution. Infection can also complicate trauma, particularly if it is associated with exposure to contaminated water such as river water or groundwater. The organism can probably penetrate an intact epithelium (Figure 3.34).

The clinical features may be quite variable. In the early phase of the disease the epithelium may be infected but not lost, so that it has a granular appearance rather than ulceration. Debridement of the epithelium may be sufficient therapy for early cases without ulceration or stromal inflammation. Even in early cases without stromal inflammation, patients can experience considerable pain (Figure 3.35). This is believed to be due to the lipases secreted by acanthamoeba, some of which resemble the pain producing elements of bee sting.

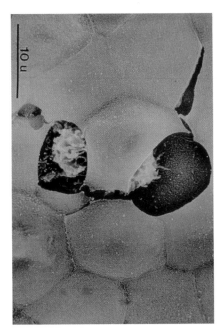

Figure 3.34 Scanning electron micrograph of acanthamoeba penetrating normal rat epithelium

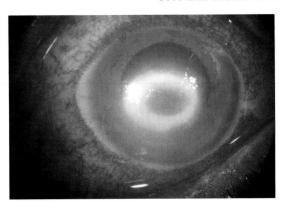

Figure 3.36 Acanthamoeba keratitis. In advanced cases a ring infiltrate can develop

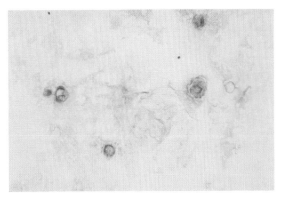

Figure 3.37 Acanthamoeba keratitis. Cysts can be seen in the smears but trophozoites are more difficult to identify

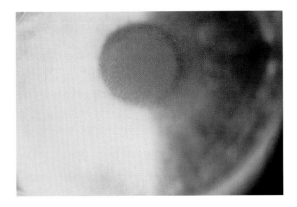

Figure 3.35 Acanthamoeba keratitis. In the earliest stages only the epithelium may be involved but the patient experiences severe pain

In more advanced cases, there is macroulceration with stromal inflammation. There is usually nothing particularly characteristic about the pattern of stromal inflammation. Sometimes, particularly in long-standing cases, there is a ring infiltrate (Figure 3.36) and sometimes the cellular infiltrate tends to occur around corneal nerves. In particularly severe cases, there may be scleral involvement.

Management involves confirming clinical suspicion by isolating the organism. Cysts but not trophozoites can be seen in a Gram stain by an experienced observer (Figure 3.37). The organism can be cultured but this may take 3–4 days. Isolation is best achieved by direct inoculation of material from the cornea onto a plain agar plate seeded with *E.coli*. Conventional scrapings are usually sufficient, but sometimes a corneal biopsy is required if the disease is progressive and scrapings have failed to yield an organism. Sometimes, although rarely now that clinicians are more experienced with the condition, the organism remains unsuspected until the patient has a corneal transplant and the

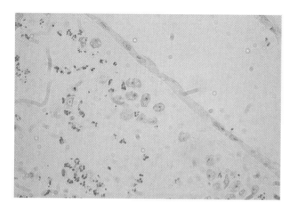

Figure 3.38 Acanthamoeba keratitis. Cysts in a cornea removed at the time of keratoplasty

Further reading

Allan BDS, Dart JKG. Strategies for the management of microbial keratitis. *Br J Ophthalmol* 1995; **79**: 777–86.

Badenoch PR, Coster DJ. Antimicrobial activity of topical anaesthetic preparations. *Br J Ophthalmol* 1982; **66**: 364.

Badenoch PR. The pathogenesis of *Acanthamoeba* keratitis. *Aust NZ J Ophthalmol* 1991; **19**: 9.

Bron AJ. A simple schema for documenting corneal disease. *Br J Ophthalmol* 1973; **57**: 629–34.

Coster DJ, Badenoch PR. Host, microbial and pharmacological factors affecting the outcome of suppurative keratitis. *Br J Ophthalmol* 1987; **71**: 96–101.

Coster DJ, Aggarwal RK, Williams KA. Surgical management of ocular surface disorders using conjunctival and stem cell allografts. *Br J Ophthalmol* 1995; **79**: 977

Coster DJ, Wilhelmus K, Peacock J, Jones BR. Suppurative keratitis in London. In: Trevor-Roper T. *The Cornea in Health and Disease*. San Diego: Academic Press, 1981.

Dart JKG. Predisposing factors in microbial keratitis: the significance of contact lens wear. *Br J Ophthalmol* 1988; **72**: 926.

Davanger M, Evensen A. Role of the pericorneal papillary structure in renewal of corneal epithelium. *Nature* 1971; **229**: 560.

DeRotth A. Plastic repair of conjunctival defects with fetal membrane. *Arch Ophthalmol* 1940; **23**: 522–5.

Goldsmith LA, Kang E, Bienfang DC *et al*. Tyrosinemia with plantar and palmar keratosis and keratitis. *J Pediatr* 1973; **83**: 798.

Gregory JK, Foster CS. Peripheral ulcerative keratitis in the collagen vascular diseases. *Int Ophthalmol Clin* 1996; **36**: 21–30.

Gundersen T. Conjunctival flaps in the treatment of corneal disease with reference to a new technique of application. *Arch Ophthalmol* 1958; **60**: 880.

Jones DB. Early diagnosis and therapy of bacterial corneal ulcers. *Int Ophthalmol Clin* 1973; **13**: 1–29.

Kirkness CM, Adams GWA, Dilly PN, Lee JP. Botulinum toxin A-induced protective ptosis in corneal disease. *Ophthalmology* 1988; **95**: 473.

O'Day DM. Selection of appropriate antifungal therapy. *Cornea* 1987; **6**: 238–45.

Ormerod LD, Gomez DS, Murphree AL *et al*. Microbial keratitis in children. *Ophthalmology* 1986; **93**: 449.

Pepose JS, Wilhelmus KR. Divergent approaches to the management of corneal ulcers. *Am J Ophthalmol* 1992; **114**: 630.

Schein OD, Ormerod LD, Barraquer E *et al*. Microbiology of contact-lens related keratitis. *Cornea* 1989; **8**: 281.

Schwartz GS, Holland EJ. Iatrogenic limbal stem cell deficiency. *Cornea* 1998; **17**: 31–7.

Stern GA. Infectious crystalline keratopathy. *Int Ophthalmol Clin* 1993; **33**: 1.

Thoft RA. Keratoepithelioplasty. *Am J Ophthalmol* 1984; **97**: 1–6.

Tseng SCG. Concept and application of limbal stem cells. *Eye* 1989; **3**: 141.

Tseng SCG, Maumenee AE, Stark WJ *et al*. Topical retinoid treatment for various dry-eye disorders. *Ophthalmology* 1985; **92**: 717.

Wood TO, Kaufman HE. Mooren's ulcer. *Am J Ophthalmol* 1971; **71**: 417.

recipient's cornea is examined histologically (Figure 3.38).

Treatment of acanthamoeba keratitis involves the use of topical anti-amoebic agents. The two most popular agents are Brolene (propamidine) and polyhexamethyl biguanide (PHMB). Either one of these agents can be used. PHMB is a little less toxic than Brolene but can be more difficult to obtain. Initial therapy involves medication four times a day. Once a satisfactory response is achieved, as judged by decreasing pain and inflammation, the frequency can be reduced to twice a day and later once a day. Both agents are toxic and when the cornea shows signs of toxicity, as judged by generalised punctate erosions, it is wise to reduce or even withdraw treatment until the signs of toxicity disappear. The drug can be recommenced when this occurs.

Topical corticosteroid may be needed to control the inflammatory response. The effect of this has not been reported other than in anecdotes, but it seems a reasonable course to take when inflammation is troublesome.

Rarely, acanthamoeba keratitis may present involving the epithelium alone. This usually occurs in contact lens wearers and is marked by epithelial opacity. Such cases have been successfully treated by epithelial debridement alone.

4 Superficial keratopathy

The superficial cornea, comprising the epithelium and the precorneal tear film it supports, has a critical role in the optimal function of the eye. Being a highly evolved and specialised structure the superficial cornea is prone to develop minor abnormalities which turn out to be clinically significant. It has evolved to serve two important but diverse functions. First, the epithelium holds the precorneal tear film which, as the anterior refracting surface of the optical system of the eye, is critical for vision. Second, it has a protective function, being the interface of the eye and the external environment. Accordingly it has developed appropriate means of reacting to challenge. This includes an ability to repair any defect promptly (the entire epithelium can be replaced in 24–48 hours) and a rich sensory innervation. Should either of the important functions be compromised symptoms arise, principally loss of vision or pain, and patients seek help. Disturbances of the corneal surface are common reasons for presentation to the ophthalmologist. Fortunately, because of the anatomical position of the corneal surface, pathological processes can be readily observed with the slit lamp, almost at a cellular level.

Common patterns of superficial keratopathy are dendritic, plaque, linear, punctate, and vortex keratopathy.

Dendritic keratopathy

Branching or dendritiform patterns in or on the corneal epithelium are easily seen with the slit lamp. They may be produced by infection with herpes simplex virus or by mucus plaques occurring in patients with herpes zoster ophthalmicus. They may also be seen in the healing phase of an acute epithelial defect. Rarely they may be seen in patients with tyrosinaemia type II.

The pathology is different in each case. The dendritic lesions seen in herpes simplex virus infection are due to the direct cytopathic effect of the virus on the epithelial cells and the spread of the virus from cell to cell (Figure 4.1). If the cytopathic effect is serious enough to cause the death and shedding of sufficient infected cells, a dendritic ulcer is formed (Figure 4.2). Otherwise, the swelling of the infected cells elevates the lesion above the plane of the surrounding cornea. The affected cells stain brilliantly with rose bengal. If there is ulceration, the exposed Bowman's membrane stains with fluorescein and the abnormal cells surrounding the ulcer stain with rose bengal (see Figure 3.16).

The dendritic figures seen in herpes zoster ophthalmicus are mucus plaques on the surface of the epithelium. Mucus aggregates on abnormal epithelium in a branching shape. There is never any ulceration unless the mucus attachment to the epithelium is so strong that a filament forms and the epithelium is stripped. This is unusual in herpes zoster ophthalmicus (Figure 4.3).

A healing abrasion is the most common cause of a dendritic lesion in the cornea. A large epithelial defect heals by sheets of epithelium sliding in from the edge. The closing edges are

Table 4.1 Patterns of superficial keratopathy and the common underlying causes

Pattern	Cause

Punctate keratopathy	Punctate epithelial erosions (non-specific lesions)
	Punctate keratopathy
	   epithelial
	   combined (stromal and epithelial)
	   stromal
	   (may be due to adenovirus, chlamydia,
	   herpes simplex virus, blepharitis, drug
	   toxicity, allograft rejection)

Dendritic keratopathy	Herpes simplex virus, herpes zoster ophthalmicus, tyrosinaemia type II, healing epithelial defect
Linear keratopathy	Fine and broad dystrophic lines Dysplasia, neoplasia Iron deposition Epithelial replacement line Epithelial rejection line
Plaque keratopathy	Mucus plaques – herpes zoster ophthalmicus Epithelial pathology Filamentary keratopathy

Vortex keratopathy	Healing epithelial defect
	Drug deposition
	   chloroquine derivatives
	   amiodarone
	Lipid deposition
	   Fabry's disease
	Melanin deposition

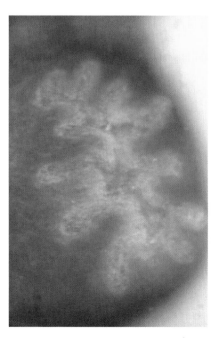

Figure 4.1 Dendritic keratitis due to herpes simplex virus infection. The virus causes a cytopathic effect in the epithelium and the cell to cell spread causes the linear branching figures

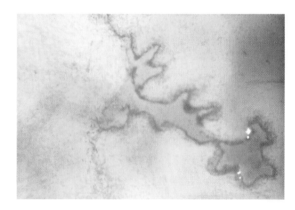

Figure 4.2 Dendritic ulceration. When the cytopathic effect is severe enough cells are shed to create a dendritic ulcer

convex and move centrally with a tangential component to their movement and when the edges meet they heap up, a little like the mountains formed when tectonic plates collide. This produces a dendritic figure which stains with rose bengal. This pattern is shortlived and lost over 48 hours (Figure 4.4; see also Figure 3.12).

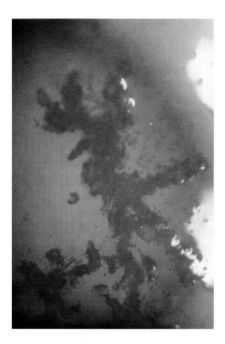

Figure 4.3   A dendritic mucus plaque in a patient with herpes zoster ophthalmicus

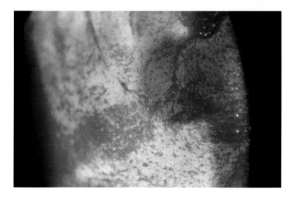

Figure 4.4   Healing epithelial defect. As the epithelial edges meet a linear branching figure is created

It is important not to confuse the various entities that can produce dendritic lesions because of the long term implications of herpes simplex virus infection. To falsely label someone as having an episode of herpetic disease may prejudice a subsequent diagnosis of corneal disease.

Plaque keratopathy

Plaques can occur when there are abnormally mucophilic patches of corneal epithelium and

mucus available in the tear film. These are aggregations of mucus on the epithelial surface. Plaques can occur in a wide range of disorders. The occurrence of dendritic plaques in herpes zoster ophthalmicus has already been discussed but other less striking small round plaques also occur in this condition and in many others (Figure 4.5). Virtually any inflammatory condition affecting the corneal epithelium can be complicated by plaque formation, including viral infections, allergic eye disease, and some disorders which are not well understood, such as superior limbic keratoconjunctivitis (Figure 4.6).

If the mucus is tenaciously attached to the epithelium, filaments may form, creating considerable discomfort or pain and a characteristic pattern of lesions. Plaques and filaments are usually seen together on the same cornea, as they are part of the same process. Filaments are composed of epithelium with adherent mucus. If enough epithelium is lifted up into the filament, corneal ulceration will occur (Figure 4.7).

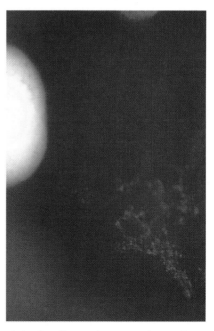

Figure 4.5   Small round mucus plaques in a patient with rubella keratitis

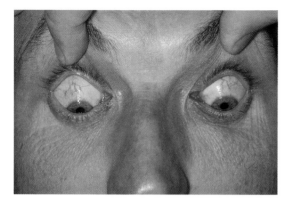

Figure 4.6 Superior limbic keratitis can be complicated by mucus plaques in the superior cornea. This may precede filament formation

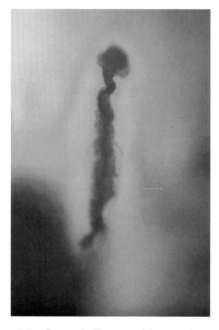

Figure 4.7 Corneal filament. Mucus plaques can lead to the development of filaments in which a tag of epithelium is elevated from the cornea

Linear keratopathy

Various lines can be seen in the cornea, some of more clinical and pathological significance than others.

Corneal lines are a prominent feature of superficial membrane dystrophies. There are two types of line seen in these dystrophies: fine lines and coarse lines. The fine lines may occur singularly or combined into arrangements that have attracted such descriptions as "mare's tail" lines. The broad lines are demarcation lines and are superficial scars formed at the edge of previous epithelial defects. These two types of line and intraepithelial microcysts are features of superficial membrane dystrophies (Figure 4.8).

Lines can form in the cornea for other reasons. Linear patterns are common in patients with dysplasia, intraepithelial carcinoma, and squamous carcinoma. Under these circumstances, a line can often be seen at the edge of the lesion, between the abnormal and normal epithelium or between two different abnormalities (Figure 4.9).

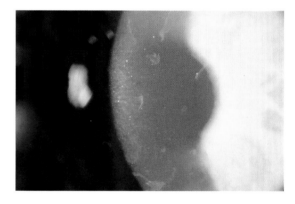

Figure 4.8 Anterior membrane dystrophy. Two types of lines are found in this condition: fine lines and broad lines. The latter are scars where the epithelium has lifted in the past

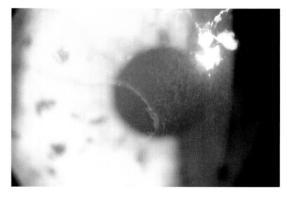

Figure 4.9 Intraepithelial neoplasia. A line can be seen between the normal and abnormal epithelium

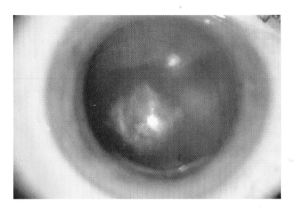

Figure 4.10 Fleischer line. Iron deposition around the base of a conical cornea

Superficial lines can also be due to deposition of material. Iron lines are common and may occur in a perfectly normal cornea, where they are described as *Hudson–Stahle* lines. Similar lines, called *Fleischer* lines (Figure 4.10), can be seen around the base of a conical cornea or around the internal edge of a pterygium where they are known as *Stocker* lines.

Linear lesions can be seen in the superficial cornea of patients who have had corneal grafts. These may be replacement lines which occur as the host epithelium pushes on to the graft to replace the donor epithelium. This process may occur a long time after the graft, even in the second or third year. Another cause of a line developing in these patients is allograft rejection directed at the corneal epithelium. It may be difficult to distinguish these two events but the best guide is the presence of inflammation, which occurs in patients undergoing rejection but not in those with replacement lines. Epithelial rejection can also produce punctate lesions in the corneal epithelium.

Superficial punctate keratopathy

Small round lesions in the superficial cornea are common, have a range of clinical appearances and can be associated with a range of disorders. These lesions may be confined to the epithelium or be in the epithelium and the superficial stroma, in which case they are known as *combined lesions*, or they may be in the superficial stroma alone. Various terms have been used to describe small round lesions in the superficial cornea and the terminology can be confusing. The terms used are descriptive clinical terms and are therefore somewhat arbitrary. Nevertheless, some consistency of description should be pursued.

Punctate epithelial erosions are very small lesions which are only seen when the cornea is stained, preferably with rose bengal. These lesions are about the size of a pin point compared to lesions described as punctate keratopathy, which are about the size of a pinhead (Figure 4.11). They have no specific pathological connotations and are found in almost all pathological processes affecting the cornea. The lesions are due to small areas of inappropriately differentiated epithelium on the

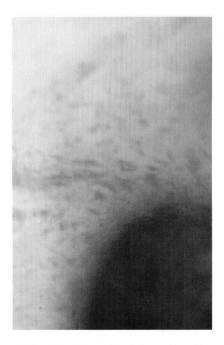

Figure 4.11 Punctate epithelial erosions. Very small lesions about the size of a pin point. They are best seen with rose bengal staining and occur in many conditions affecting the ocular surface

corneal surface. This may occur with epithelial wound healing, toxicity, dysplasia, and neoplasia or with disturbances in the outer eye associated with abnormal nutrition. Punctate epithelial erosions are the tiny staining lesions seen when the corneas of patients with dry eyes are stained with rose bengal.

Superficial punctate keratopathy is the term used to describe "spotty" lesions in the superficial cornea. These lesions occur in a number of circumstances and are about the size of a pinhead. They are nests of abnormal epithelial cells (Figure 4.12).

The conditions in which they occur include adenoviral keratoconjunctivitis, chlamydial keratoconjunctivitis, vaccinial infection, herpes simplex virus infection, blepharokeratoconjunctivitis, allograft rejection, and Thygeson's superficial punctate keratopathy.

The lesions may be epithelial, involve the epithelium and the superficial stroma or just the superficial stroma. Typically, in cases of adenoviral keratoconjunctivitis the lesions are initially epithelial, then the stroma becomes involved and over weeks the epithelial pathology regresses until only the stromal opacity can be seen (Figure 4.13). When the stromal lesions are large the condition is described as *nummular keratitis* (Figure 4.14).

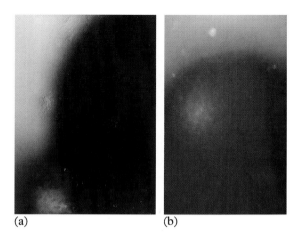

(a)   (b)

Figure 4.13 Superficial punctate keratopathy. When part of adenoviral keratoconjunctivitis, the lesions are initially small and confined to the epithelium (a) and later the stroma is involved and the epithelium heals (b)

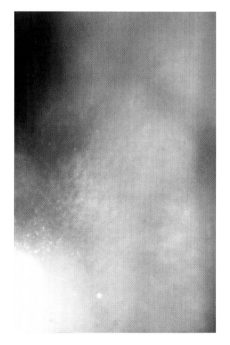

Figure 4.14 Nummular keratitis. Large round lesions of inflammation and later scarring in the superficial corneal stroma

Diagnosis

A few well directed enquiries will establish the cause of superficial punctate keratopathy. A systemic approach to identify the various causes of punctate keratopathy is required.

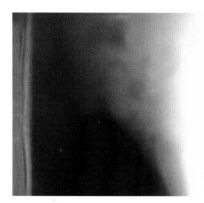

Figure 4.12 Superficial punctate keratopathy. These "nests" of abnormal cells are about the size of a pinhead. They occur in a wide range of corneal disorders

First, the state of the eyelids must be considered. If there is significant blepharitis, this may be the cause of the keratopathy. Lid vesicles suggest the possibility of herpes simplex virus infection. Similarly blepharitis may be associated with punctate keratopathy and molluscum contagiosum will cause a similar picture.

If the lids are normal the conjunctiva must then be assessed to see if it is abnormal. If there is a follicular conjunctivitis, then the keratopathy may be due to infection with herpes simplex virus as a primary infection, adenovirus, or chlamydia. There may be features in the conjunctival reaction which suggest the aetiological agent. For example, an acute follicular reaction with subconjunctival haemorrhage suggests infection with adenovirus.

A more chronic form of follicular conjunctivitis (with a history of more than three weeks' duration) suggests chlamydial infection. If there are lid vesicles and an acute follicular conjunctivitis in a young person with superficial punctate keratopathy, a primary infection with herpes simplex virus is the likely cause.

If the lids and the conjunctiva are normal, the lesions could be due to Thygeson's superficial punctate keratopathy. This is a condition of unknown cause. Various viruses and immunological processes have been suggested, but not confirmed, as causes. The condition presents with photophobia and superficial punctate keratopathy. It affects young and middle aged men and women and runs a relapsing and recurrent course. The corneal lesions are small, like bread crumbs, and entirely confined to the epithelium. Another characteristic feature is that the condition is usually sensitive to steroids, which relieve symptoms and reduce or eradicate lesions within days. Patients presenting with superficial keratopathy and with lesions confined entirely to the epithelium and with no evidence of lid or conjunctival disease should be suspected of having Thygeson's disease. Two further issues need to be resolved to confirm the clinical suspicion.

Is the course of the disease relapsing? To assess this, the patient must be observed over a period of time; this can be resolved by withholding treatment and charting the course or by treating the presenting attack and then withdrawing treatment and observing for recurrences.

Is the process sensitive to topical steroids? Most cases of Thygeson's disease respond promptly to topical corticosteroids with abatement of symptoms and resolution of lesions. A trial of treatment, prednisolone phosphate 0.5% eye drops four times a day for a week, is an appropriate therapeutic trial. This approach to diagnosis is summarised in Figures 4.15 and 4.16.

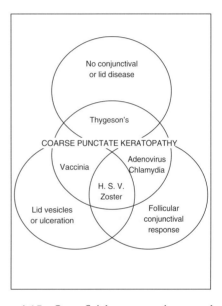

Figure 4.15 Superficial punctate keratopathy. The relationship of punctate keratopathy to lid and conjunctival disease

Vortex keratopathy

A common pattern of change in the superficial cornea is a swirling pattern in the epithelium, like water going down a plug hole. For this to occur, something must opacify the corneal epithelium and this opacification makes the migration of the epithelium visible. Normally the epithelium is generated deep in the limbus and as the cells divide and mature, they move centrally, tangentially, and become more superficial, reaching their terminal differentiation on the

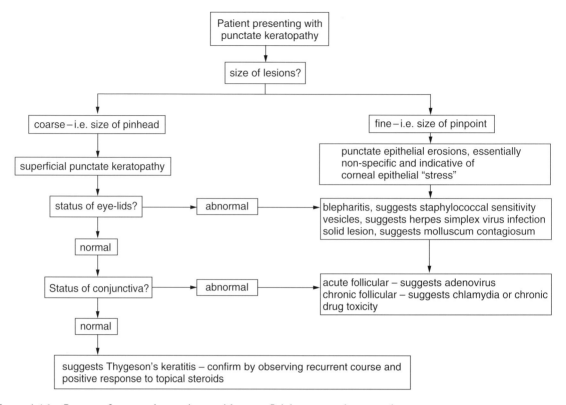

```
                    ┌─────────────────────┐
                    │ Patient presenting with │
                    │ punctate keratopathy │
                    └─────────────────────┘
                              │
                    ┌─────────────────┐
                    │ size of lesions? │
                    └─────────────────┘
```

coarse – i.e. size of pinhead

fine – i.e. size of pinpoint

superficial punctate keratopathy

punctate epithelial erosions, essentially non-specific and indicative of corneal epithelial "stress"

status of eye-lids? → abnormal

blepharitis, suggests staphylococcal sensitivity
vesicles, suggests herpes simplex virus infection
solid lesion, suggests molluscum contagiosum

normal

Status of conjunctiva? → abnormal

acute follicular – suggests adenovirus
chronic follicular – suggests chlamydia or chronic drug toxicity

normal

suggests Thygeson's keratitis – confirm by observing recurrent course and positive response to topical steroids

Figure 4.16 Strategy for assessing patients with superficial punctate keratopathy

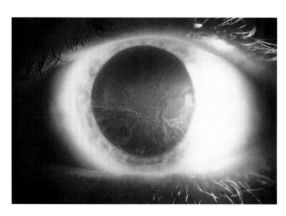

Figure 4.17 Vortex keratopathy in a patient receiving amiodarone

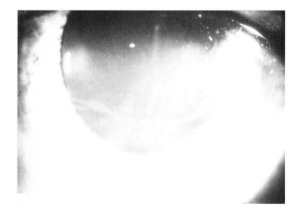

Figure 4.18 Vortex keratopathy in a patient with Fabry's disease

central corneal surface. The epithelium can be marked by drug deposition, as occurs with chloroquine derivatives and amiodarone (Figure 4.17), and by lipid deposition, as occurs in Fabry's disease (Figure 4.18). Sometimes, in deeply pigmented patients, cells from the limbus containing melanin produce the same pattern.

Further reading

Burns RP, Gipson IK, Murray MJ. Keratopathy in tyrosinemia. *Birth Defects* 1976; **12**: 169.

Ford E, Nelson KE, Warren D. Epidemiology of epidemic keratoconjuctivitis. *Epidemiol Rev* 1987; **9**: 244.

Foster CS. Cicatricial pemphigoid. *Trans Am Ophthalmol Soc* 1986; **84**: 527.

Fraunfelder FT, Wright P, Tripathi RC. Corneal mucus plaques. *Am J Ophthalmol* 1977; **83**: 191.

Hoang-Xuan T, Rodriguez A, Zaltas MM, Rice BA, Foster CS. Ocular rosacea: a histologic and immunopathologic study. *Ophthalmology* 1990; **97**: 1468–75.

Jones BR. The differential diagnosis of punctate keratitis. *Trans Ophthalmol Soc UK* 1961; **80**: 655.

Jones DB. Prospects in the management of tear-deficient states. *Trans Am Acad Ophthalmol Otolaryngol* 1977; **83**: 693.

Kaden I, Mayers M. Systemic associations of dry-eye syndrome. *Int Ophthalmol Clin* 1991; **31**: 69.

Kaufman HE. Keratitis sicca. *Int Ophthalmol Clin* 1984; **24**: 133.

Kenyon KR. *Anatomy and Pathology of the Ocular Surface*. Boston: Little, Brown, 1979.

McCulley JP, Dougherty J. Classification of chronic blepharitis. *Ophthalmology* 1982; **89**: 1173.

Nichols BA, Chiappino ML, Dawson CR. Demonstration of the mucous layer of the tear film by electron microscopy. *Invest Ophthalmol Vis Sci* 1985; **26**: 464.

Shine WE, McCulley JP. Keratoconjunctivitis sicca associated with meibomian secretion polar lipid abnormality. *Arch Ophthalmol* 1998; **116**: 849–52.

Sjögren H, Block KK. Keratoconjunctivitis sicca and the Sjögren syndrome. *Surv Ophthalmol* 1971; **16**: 145.

Stevens AJ. The meibomian secretions. *Int Ophthalmol Clin* 1938; **13**: 159.

Sullivan HH, Beard C, Bullock JD. Cryosurgery for the treatment of trichiasis. *Ophthalmic Surg* 1977; **10**: 42.

Theodore FH, Ferry AP. Superior limbic keratoconjunctivitis. Clinical and pathological correlations. *Arch Ophthalmol* 1970; **84**: 481.

Thygeson P. Complications of staphylococcic blepharitis. *Am J Ophthalmol* 1969; **68**: 446.

Thygeson P. Superficial punctate keratitis. *JAMA* 1950; **144**: 1544.

Thygeson P, Kimura SJ. Chronic conjunctivitis. *Trans Am Acad Ophthalmol Otolaryngol* 1963; **67**: 494.

Zaidman GW, Geeraets R, Paylor RR, Ferry AP. The histopathology of filamentary keratitis. *Arch Ophthalmol* 1985; **103**: 1178.

5 Corneal complications of contact lens wear

Contact lens wear is common. For the most part, contact lenses are highly successful devices but complications are relatively common although, fortunately, most are not threatening. They arise because a relatively large prosthetic device is imposed on the delicate ecosystem of the external eye. Although complications occur frequently, it is important to remember that not all corneal disease in contact lens wearers results from the lens. There may be a corneal disorder which has provided the indication for contact lens use in the first place or there may be coincidental disease. Conjunctivitis, keratitis and blepharitis, and all other corneal disorders that occur in non-contact lens wearers occur in those who use the devices. This means that any assessment of corneal disorders in patients who use contact lenses must be extensive enough to look not only for the complications of contact lens use but also for other conditions which affect the outer eye.

The most important complications of contact lens use are corneal infections. It is important to recognise the possibility of acute corneal infection as a cause of ocular inflammation in contact lens wearers and to investigate and treat the condition as the emergency it is. Even though this is one of the less common complications of contact lens wear it should be given precedence in the diagnostic process and raised as a hypothesis early on, because it is the most serious complication of contact lens wear.

Contact lens wear and the ocular surface ecosystem

Contact lenses can have a disturbing impact on the fragile corneal ecosystem and can affect all elements of the system (Figure 5.1). Their presence on the cornea may alter the epithelium and the stroma and even the endothelium. Of critical importance is the impact they have on the epithelium, which may be minor, in the form of microcysts, or more serious, through various mechanisms which may lead to corneal ulceration. Contact lens wear may also affect the conjunctiva. As a foreign body which may accumulate proteins and other biomaterial on its surface, the contact lens may initiate immunological or toxic reactions which will be manifested in conjunctival changes. Lenses can

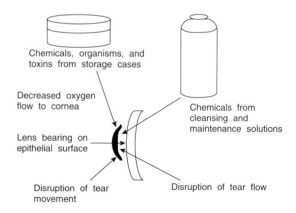

Figure 5.1 Impact of contact lens wear on the ecosystem of the cornea and ocular surface

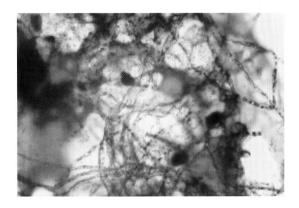

Figure 5.2 Gram stain of the contents of a contact lens case belonging to a patient presenting with ocular inflammation. Numerous bacteria, fungi, and acanthamoeba were found in the case

carry toxic material, such as preservatives and other chemicals used in lens maintenance, which may prove to be toxic when exposed to the conjunctiva. The lens may function as a reservoir for the slow but constant release of toxins into the conjunctival sac. Contact lenses will also alter the normal pattern of tear flow which, in extreme cases, may lead to corneal anoxia. Similarly, they may affect normal blinking patterns.

When not in the eye, contact lenses live in a watery environment which inevitably carries its own bio-burden and the weight of this burden is evident from studies looking at the "normal flora" of contact lens cases and solutions. Large numbers of waterborne micro-organisms may be present in inadequately maintained cases (Figure 5.2) or on the lenses. Simply washing the lens with tap water may provide significant numbers of organisms capable of serious disease, such as acanthamoeba, when the lens is placed on the eye.

Despite the environmental threat to the outer eye which can be posed by contact lenses, complications are relatively few and almost all, apart from microbial keratitis, can be reversed simply by refraining from lens use until the problem is resolved.

A diagnostic approach to the complications of contact lens wear

When faced with a corneal disorder in a patient who is a contact lens wearer, there are three questions which should be answered in the diagnostic decision making process. The first question is whether the eye is inflamed. If the eye is inflamed, the next question is whether the inflammation is primarily in the conjunctiva or in the cornea. The third question is whether there is acute stromal inflammation.

If the eye is inflamed, a focus of inflammation with a dense stromal cellular infiltrate, approaching that of abscess formation, suggests the serious possibility of infection. If the cornea is relatively unaffected and the inflammatory process is mainly in the conjunctiva, then the most likely possibility is either papillary conjunctivitis or a sensitivity reaction to the lens or solutions. If the cornea is primarily involved and there is only a surrounding response in the conjunctiva of minor degree, then the pathology is probably confined to the epithelium which may be damaged by abrasion or hypoxia or, if the condition is more chronic, by toxic changes from the lens or the solutions used to maintain it. If there is the serious complication of stromal infiltration, then the state of the epithelium is of prime concern. If there is corneal ulceration and stromal suppuration, then infection should be considered present until proven otherwise. If, on the other hand, the cellular infiltrates are small, single or multiple but tending towards the periphery of the cornea with an overlying intact epithelium, they may be sterile and can be safely observed over 24 hours, after removal of the lens. If the epithelium is intact, it is usually best to avoid scraping of the cornea for the collection of material for microbiology assessment and so avoid further damage to a fragile but intact epithelium. An algorithm for approaching ocular inflammation in a contact lens wearer is set out in Figure 5.3.

If the eye is not inflamed, the first question to ask is whether there has been any visual loss. If there is visual loss, it may be due to epithelial oedema, stromal oedema, corneal warpage, or limbal dysplasia creating opaque epithelium. If there is no visual loss, then the changes in the cornea must be more limited, with epithelial

CORNEA

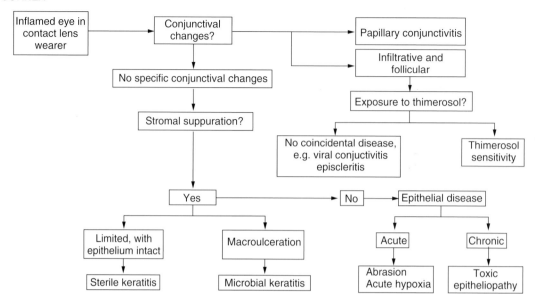

Figure 5.3   Algorithm for clinical diagnosis in patients with ocular inflammation who wear contact lenses

microcysts, perhaps stromal neovascularisation or endothelial polymegathism. An algorithm for assessing patients with non-inflammatory complications of contact lens wear is set out in Figure 5.4.

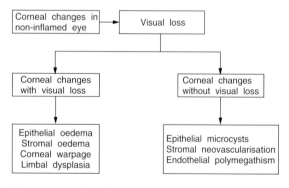

Figure 5.4   Algorithm for the assessment of patients with non-inflammatory complications of contact lens wear

Inflammatory complications of contact lens wear

Microbial keratitis

Patients wearing contact lenses are at increased risk of corneal infection. The presence of a contact lens compromises the ocular surface and alters the pattern of organisms in the conjunctival sac. Anyone wearing a contact lens who has an epithelial defect and a corneal inflammatory cell infiltrate should be considered to have infection until proven otherwise.

The management of microbial keratitis in contact lens wearers is the same as for anyone else. The lens should be removed, microbiological investigations carried out, and antimicrobial chemotherapy commenced. Management details are set out in the section dealing with microbial keratitis in Chapter 3.

The pattern of causal organisms is slightly different in contact lens wearers. There are relatively more Gram negative organisms, which reflects the alteration in commensal populations in contact lens wearers which, in turn, is due to the watery extraocular environment in which contact lenses are maintained. For the same reason, contact lens wearers are more susceptible to acanthamoeba keratitis (Figure 5.5).

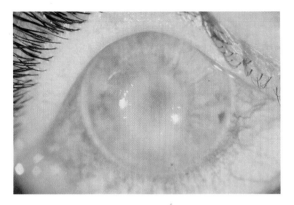

Figure 5.5 Acanthamoeba keratitis complicating contact lens wear

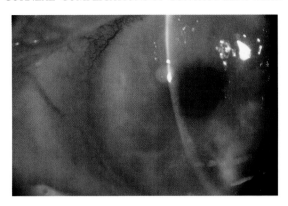

Figure 5.7 Acute epitheliopathy related to contact lens wear. A small area of necrosis and ulceration has developed in an area of oedema

Sterile infiltrative keratitis

Contact lens wearers are prone to develop small cellular infiltrates in the corneal stroma. They can occur as solitary or multiple lesions and may be so dense as to be considered abscesses. They tend to be peripheral and the epithelium over the lesions is often intact. If the infiltrate is large and superficial, the epithelium may break down over the lesion (Figure 5.6).

The cause of these lesions is not proven. A number of factors could account for white cell recruitment through limbal vessels into the cornea, but the most likely reason is the presence of foreign proteins such as bacterial endotoxins which are potent promoters of white cell recruitment.

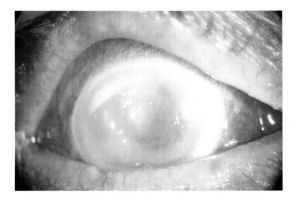

Figure 5.6 Sterile corneal infiltrate in a cornea which has become oedematous under a contact lens. No organism was detected and the cornea quickly settled with the lens removed

The treatment of patients with these lesions consists of removal of the lens and observation over 24 hours, unless suspicion of infection is high. If the epithelium is deficient and suspicion of infection is high, then the pathology should be ascribed to microbial infection until proven otherwise.

Acute epitheliopathy

Patients wearing contact lenses may suddenly develop inflammation; the only pathology detectable is an abnormality in the epithelium which may be a small area of necrosis or ulceration. This picture may be due to hypoxia, when it is usually more widespread, or it may be due to an abrasion as a consequence of an inappropriate lens shape or a small foreign body under the lens (Figure 5.7).

Chronic toxic corneal epitheliopathy

A form of epitheliopathy which is more chronic may be due to toxins in the lens or in the chemicals the lens brings to the eye. In such cases, the conjunctival changes are less marked but with some vascular injection. The changes seen in the cornea are principally multiple punctate epithelial erosions or even punctate keratopathy (Figure 5.8).

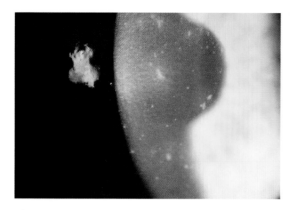

Figure 5.8 Toxic corneal epitheliopathy with widespread punctate epithelial erosions and punctate keratopathy

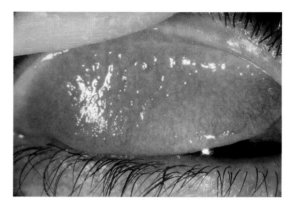

Figure 5.9 Giant papillary conjunctivitis. Patients usually present with diffuse conjunctival thickening and only the beginnings of papillae formation

Papillary conjunctivitis

If the inflammation is primarily conjunctival, the most likely diagnosis is papillary conjunctivitis. This can occur in all lens wearers but is more common in patients wearing soft lenses and can occur in patients not wearing lenses at all if they have had surgery and there is a nylon suture exposed on the ocular surface. Those affected experience ocular inflammation, particularly when wearing the lenses, and may experience excessive mucus secretion. Sometimes the earliest symptom is increased mobility of the lens on the eye. Usually the condition develops some time after successful contact lens wear has been established. Examination reveals minimal corneal changes but there may be some punctate epithelial erosions, a conjunctivitis in which the mucosa is thickened and oedematous (Figure 5.9), and where the submucosal thickening is organised into papillae. Patients usually present when the conjunctival signs are mild. It is unusual to see the disease progress to giant papillae, the sign after which the condition is named (Figure 5.10).

The condition is believed to be due to the development of an allergic response either to the lens or to proteins collecting on the lens.

The general approach to treatment is to carefully check the lens care arrangements and to ensure that they are optimal. Any spoiled lens

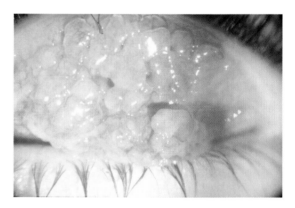

Figure 5.10 Giant papillary conjunctivitis. Gross papillae development is unusual today

should be changed, perhaps to an alternative form of lens. For example, a soft lens may be changed to a semi-rigid gas permeable lens. If these measures fail, topical steroids should be considered along with limiting the duration of contact lens wear.

Chronic allergic conjunctivitis: thimerosol allergy

This condition is much less common than in the past because there is an increased awareness of the toxic effects of the chemicals used in contact lens maintenance and because thimerosol has been largely replaced in contact lens care solutions.

Some patients are very sensitive to preservatives and develop a toxic conjunctivitis.

Table 5.1 Summary of inflammatory complications of contact lens wear

Inflammation	Agent	Inflamed eye	Corneal signs	Conjunctival signs
Suppurative keratitis	Microbial keratitis	Intense inflammation	Ulceration Cellular infiltrate Oedema Anterior chamber reaction	Intense injection
	Sterile keratitis	Mild to moderate	Usually peripheral May or may not be ulcerated Small infiltrate(s)	Moderate injection No specific signs
Epitheliopathy	Corneal abrasion	Moderate to severe with severe pain	Macroulceration No stromal inflammation	Moderate injection No specific signs
	Acute hypoxic epitheliopathy	Mild to moderate	Punctate epithelial erosions usually central, sometimes with epithelial loss	Moderate injection No specific signs
	Toxic epitheliopathy	Mild to moderate Maximal after lens insertion	Punctate epithelial erosions Punctate keratopathy	Moderate infection No specific signs
	Thimerosol allergy	Inflammation with lens wear	Punctate epithe lial erosions and punctate epitheliopathy, particularly in superior cornea	Superior limbal infection, thickened conjunctiva, sometimes with follicles
Conjunctivitis	Papillary conjunctivitis	Mild to moderate inflammation when wearing lenses	Usually none	Infection with papillary changes

These patients experience mild to moderate inflammation of the eyes which is maximal after lens insertion. The cornea shows punctate epithelial erosions and sometimes shows punctate keratopathy but, although the conjunctiva is inflamed, there are no specific signs attributable to this type of conjunctivitis. A summary of the inflammatory changes which can occur in contact lens wearers is set out in Table 5.1.

Non-inflammatory complications of contact lens wear

Contact lens wear can cause non-inflammatory complications. Sometimes these changes are associated with visual loss and sometimes not. If there is no inflammation or visual loss, the changes are asymptomatic and tend to be found on routine examination. Of those that affect vision

adversely, oedema, corneal warpage, and limbal dysplasia are the most serious.

Oedema

Corneal oedema occurs when contact lens wear interferes with the normal corneal physiology.

If the lens, for whatever reason, reduces the amount of oxygen available to the cornea, the metabolically active pump required to keep the cornea relatively dry fails and the corneal stroma and epithelium become oedematous. This is always associated with impaired vision. If the oedema is prolonged, it may be complicated by neovascularisation and inflammation. The corneal epithelium depends on tear flow for nutrition and oxygenation and this may be reduced under a contact lens. Acute hypoxia may result, leading to epithelial oedema and even epithelial necrosis without stromal oedema.

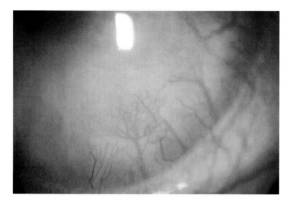

Figure 5.11   Contact lens induced corneal oedema with subsequent stromal neovascularisation

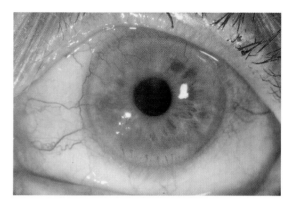

Figure 5.12   Limbal dysplasia in a young contact lens wearer

Even when severe, oedema is not usually associated with inflammation unless there is epithelial damage, but if the oedema is prolonged there may be sufficient disruption of corneal tissues to induce inflammation and neovascularisation (Figure 5.11).

Corneal hypoxia and corneal oedema are serious threats to the long term integrity of the cornea and must be dealt with promptly. Contact lens wear should be stopped and the clinical situation reviewed, with the intention of finding a better contact lens arrangement for the patient. Corneal oedema from contact lenses is quite rare in patients who are using modern lenses and following the recommended care regimens.

Corneal warpage

Patients wearing contact lenses may develop irregular corneal astigmatism due to changes in the corneal stroma. These changes tend to be insignificant while the patient is wearing the contact lens but when the lens is removed the best corrected vision is found to have dropped, a situation originally described as "spectacle blur". The cause is unknown and, again, the condition is uncommon with modern lenses.

Limbal dysplasia

Patients wearing contact lenses can develop abnormalities of the limbal epithelium which may involve the cornea. The condition which arises is indistinguishable from the limbal dysplasia associated with long term exposure to high levels of ultraviolet light, but neoplastic change has not been recorded in such cases. The limbal epithelium becomes opaque and this may extend into the cornea. Often there is associated superficial vascularisation (Figure 5.12).

This condition represents a serious threat to the integrity of the normal corneal epithelium and has serious consequences for vision. For these reasons, patients developing limbal dysplasia should be discouraged from continuing contact lens wear.

Epithelial microcysts

Epithelial microcysts are commonly found in contact lens wearers, especially in patients who are long term contact lens wearers. Presumably they occur as a consequence of irritation of the epithelium which bears the contact lens. They are seldom of any significance (Figure 5.13).

Endothelial polymegathism

Irregularity in the size and shape of the endothelium develops in long term contact lens wearers. It has been assumed that this is associated with reduced endothelial cell functional reserve capacity, but this has never been reported to be a clinical problem. It has been suggested that patients with polymegathism are at increased risk from intraocular surgery but this has not been confirmed either.

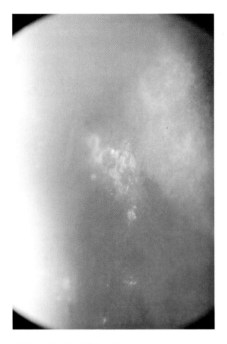

Figure 5.13   Epithelial microcysts in a contact lens wearer

The condition is a curiosity rather than an important clinical entity.

Corneal neovascularisation

There are two forms of corneal neovascularisation associated with contact lens wear. The most serious is deep stromal neovascularisation which is invariably associated with chronic stromal oedema (see Figure 5.11). The second is superficial subepithelial neovascularisation which can occur for a number of reasons but which is usually associated with chronic irritation of the corneal epithelium. It occurs in patients who are prone to ocular surface inflammation, such as those who are atopic.

Corneal neovascularisation is a serious complication of contact lens wear. It can be associated with lipid deposition which is difficult to treat and which adversely affects vision. Invariably, neovascularisation is associated with increased numbers of inflammatory cells in the cornea and their presence worsens the prognosis for corneal

Table 5.2   Summary of the non-inflammatory corneal complications of contact lens wear

Corneal changes	Inflammation	Corneal signs	Conjunctival signs
Epithelial Microcystic keratopathy	None	Epithelial microcysts No stromal changes	None
Epithelial oedema	None	Epithelial oedema	None
Limbal dysplasia	None	Epithelial opacity linked to limbus	None

Stroma
  Stromal oedema
	None	Epithelial oedema
		   in advanced cells
		Stromal oedema,
		   often with folds
			None

Neovascularisation	None	Neovascularisation can occur at any level, sometimes associated with oedema	None
Corneal warpage	None	Irregular astigmatism No morphological changes	None

Endothelial
  Polymegathism
	None	Variable shape and size
		   of endothelial cells
			None

transplantation should this ever be required. The stromal form of neovascularisation is more of a threat to the cornea than superficial vascularisation which, once established, is not progressive so that the condition is not necessarily a contraindication to contact lens wear. A summary of the non-inflammatory corneal disorders associated with contact lens wear is set out in Table 5.2.

Further reading

Allansmith MR, Korb DR, Greiner JV. Giant papillary conjunctivitis induced by hard or soft contact lens wear: quantitative histology. *Ophthalmology* 1978; **85**: 766–78.

Binda PS, Rasmussen DM, Gordon M. Keratoconjunctivitis and soft contact lens solutions. *Arch Ophthalmol* 1981; **99**: 87.

Bloomfield SE, Jakobiec FA, Theodore FH. Contact lens induced keratopathy: a severe complication extending the spectrum of keratoconjunctivitis in contact lens wearers. *Ophthalmology* 1984; **91**: 290.

Cheng KH, Leung SL, Hoekman HW *et al.* Incidence of contact-lens-associated microbial keratitis and its related morbidity. *Lancet* 1999; **354**: 181–5.

Gordon A, Kracher GP. Corneal infiltrates and extended-wear contact lenses. *J Am Optom Assoc* 1985; **56**: 198–201.

Grant T, Chong MS, Vajdic C *et al.* Contact lens induced peripheral ulcers during hydrogel contact lens wear. *CLAO J* 1998; **24**: 145–51.

Gudmundsson OG, Ormerod LD, Kenyon KR *et al.* Factors influencing predilection and outcome of bacterial keratitis. *Cornea* 1989; **8**: 115.

Holden BA, Vannas A, Nilsson LK *et al.* Epithelial and endothelial effects from the extended wear of contact lenses. The effects of contact lenses on the normal physiology and anatomy of the cornea: symposium summary. *Curr Eye Res* 1985; **4**: 739.

Josephson JE, Caffery BE. Proposed hypothesis for corneal infiltrates, microabrasions, and red eye associated with extended wear (letter). *Optom Vis Sci* 1989; **66**: 192.

MacRae SM, Matsuda M, Shellans S, Rich LF. The effects of hard and soft contact lenses on the corneal endothelium. *Am J Ophthalmol* 1986; **102**: 50.

Mondino BJ, Groden LR. Conjunctival hyperemia and corneal infiltrates with chemically disinfected soft contact lenses. *Arch Ophthalmol* 1980; **98**: 1767.

Poggio EC, Glynn RJ, Schein OD *et al.* The incidence of ulcerative keratitis among users of daily-wear and extended-wear soft contact lenses. *N Engl J Med* 1989; **321**: 779.

Polse KA, Brand RJ, Cohen SR, Guillon M. Hypoxic effects on corneal morphology and function. *Invest Ophthalmol Vis Sci* 1990; **31**: 1542–54.

Ruben M. Acute eye disease secondary to contact-lens wear. Report of a census. *Lancet* 1976; **1**: 138.

Schein OD, Glynn RJ, Poggio EC *et al.* The relative risk of ulcerative keratitis among users of daily-wear and extended-wear soft contact lenses: a case-control study. *N Engl J Med* 1989; **321**: 773.

Schein OD, Ormerod LD, Barraquer E *et al.* Microbiology of contact-lens related keratitis. *Cornea* 1989; **8**: 281.

Schoessler JP, Orsborn GN. A theory of corneal endothelial polymegathism and aging. *Curr Eye Res* 1987; **6**: 301.

Stein RM, Clinch TE, Cohen EJ *et al.* Infected vs sterile corneal infiltrates in contact lens wearers. *Am J Ophthalmol* 1988; **105**: 632.

Stenson S. Superior limbic keratoconjunctivitis associated with soft contact lens wear. *Arch Ophthalmol* 1983; **101**: 402–4.

6 Interstitial keratitis

Interstitial keratitis is a term used to describe inflammation of the corneal stroma without epithelial loss. It was originally used by Hutchinson in the 1850s to describe corneal opacification associated with syphilis. Although there are many other causes of non-ulcerative stromal inflammation recognised today, syphilis remains an important cause and should be foremost in the clinician's mind when dealing with patients with interstitial keratitis because of the sinister implications for general health.

Clinical features

Patients presenting with interstitial keratitis have decreased vision, discomfort, if the inflammation is at all severe, and photophobia.

Examination reveals evidence of ocular injection in all but the mildest cases and the focus of inflammation is in the corneal stroma and may take distinct forms. Acute inflammation may be so intense as to cause suppuration or it may be less intense with cellular infiltration and oedema, which may be focal, multifocal, or diffuse.

The clinician needs to identify the pattern of inflammation. Suppuration with an intact epithelium is most often due to herpes simplex virus infection but can be due to infection with a relatively non-virulent micro-organism. Bacteria, such as those responsible for infectious crystalline keratopathy, and some fungi can find their way through an apparently intact corneal epithelium to establish stromal infection.

Non-suppurative inflammation, either single focus or diffuse, may be due to infection with herpes simplex virus, varicella-zoster virus, Epstein–Barr virus, acanthamoeba, syphilis, or leprosy or may be due to conditions of unknown aetiology, such as sarcoidosis or Cogan's syndrome.

Multifocal inflammation may be due to viral infection with herpes simplex virus, adenovirus, or Epstein–Barr virus or may be associated with contact lens wear. When the inflammatory lesions are flat and relatively large, more than 0.5 mm in diameter, the term *nummular keratitis* is sometimes used. A similar picture can be seen after blunt trauma to the eye, in which case the opacities are not inflammatory but oedematous, resulting from focal endothelial damage.

Causes of interstitial keratitis

The causes of interstitial keratitis are set out in Box 6.1 and an algorithm for diagnosis is shown in Figure 6.1. Herpes simplex virus infection is the most common cause of interstitial keratitis in most urban societies but syphilis is the most important diagnosis, for the reasons mentioned above.

Herpes simplex virus stromal keratitis

This is the most common cause of interstitial keratitis in Western urban societies. Several distinct patterns occur. Inflammation due to herpes simplex virus may be non-suppurative or

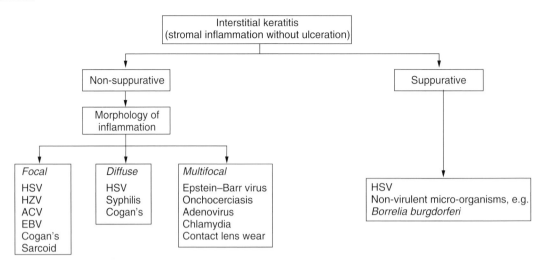

Figure 6.1 Algorithm for diagnosis of interstitial keratitis

Box 6.1 *Causes of interstitial keratitis*

Viruses	Herpes simplex virus
	Varicella–zoster virus
	Epstein–Barr virus
	Adenovirus
	Mumps virus
Bacteria	*Treponema pallidum*
	Mycobacterial tubercle
	Mycobacterium leprae
	Lyme disease
Chlamydia	
Parasitic diseases	Onchocerciasis
	Trypsomiasis
	Leishmaniasis
	Malaria
	Acanthamoeba
	Cysticercosis
Unknown causes	Cogan's syndrome
	Mycosis fungoides
	Sarcoidosis

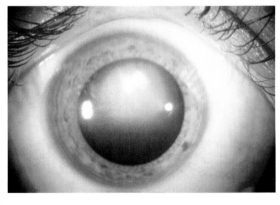

Figure 6.2 Disciform interstitial keratitis. Herpes simplex virus infection is the usual cause

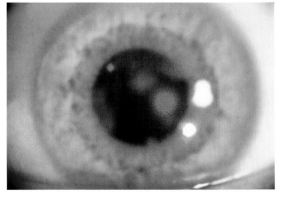

Figure 6.3 Multifocal disciform keratitis due to herpes simplex virus infection

suppurative. The non-suppurative form may be disciform (oval) (Figure 6.2), usually with one area of inflammation, but less commonly may be multifocal (Figure 6.3). It can also be diffuse. The pathology is not fully understood but it is believed to be due to the host response to viral antigens. Often there is an associated anterior uveitis and quite often the intraocular pressure is raised.

Suppurative or necrotising stromal keratitis may occur in association with corneal ulceration and can be severe, particularly in recurrent cases, beneath an intact epithelium. There is usually an associated uveitis which may be severe enough to create a hypopyon. It is characteristic of herpetic stromal keratitis that the anterior chamber reaction is commensurate with the degree of inflammation in the cornea. Bacterial keratitis, on the other hand, tends to create an anterior chamber reaction which exceeds the level of inflammation in the stroma. Nevertheless, it is impossible to clinically differentiate with any degree of certainty between corneal ulceration with stromal necrosis caused by herpes simplex virus infection and that due to bacterial infection.

At present there is no laboratory test which can be used to confirm herpes simplex virus as the cause of interstitial keratitis.

Treatment is aimed at suppressing stromal inflammation with topical corticosteroids without exposing the epithelium to the risks of herpetic infection and ulceration. This requires the use of topical antiviral cover.

Epstein–Barr virus (mononucleosis) interstitial keratitis

Interstitial keratitis can complicate infectious mononucleosis syndrome (glandular fever). Early on in the illness, patients develop a multifocal stromal keratitis. This may be superficial, mid-stromal or deep. The epithelium is not usually affected. When the lesions are subepithelial, they resemble those seen late in the course of adenoviral keratoconjunctivitis. The systemic disorder may last weeks or months but the stromal changes may last for years (Figure 6.4).

Other ocular complications of Epstein–Barr infection include conjunctivitis with preauricular lymphadenitis (oculoglandular syndrome) and dacroadenitis.

Serological support for a clinical diagnosis is compelling. IgM and IgG increase within weeks,

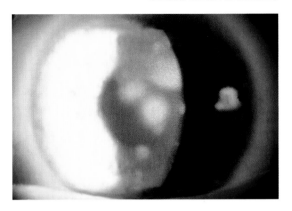

Figure 6.4 Multifocal interstitial keratitis due to Epstein–Barr virus infection

the IgM falling within six months but IgG remaining detectable throughout life.

Treatment involves use of topical corticosteroids when patients are troubled by symptoms or when corneal neovascularisation complicates stromal inflammation. Antiviral chemotherapy is of no proven value.

Varicella-zoster interstitial keratitis

Inflammation of the corneal stroma is a rare complication of chickenpox but a common complication of herpes zoster ophthalmicus.

Both non-suppurative and suppurative inflammation occurs. Non-suppurative stromal keratitis is the most common form of the disease

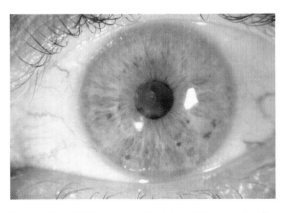

Figure 6.5 Diffuse interstitial keratitis complicating herpes zoster ophthalmicus

and may be focal, with single or multiple oval (disciform) lesions, or diffuse (Figure 6.5). Epithelial pathology, including ulceration, is not part of the problem. Often there is anterior chamber reaction and sometimes ocular inflammation. Chronicity is a common problem which can lead to stromal neovascularisation and lipid deposition.

Treatment is aimed at suppressing corneal inflammation with topical corticosteroids. There is no indication for antiviral chemotherapy. If there is accompanying scleral inflammation, oral corticosteroids may be necessary to decrease pain and minimise the risk of tissue damage.

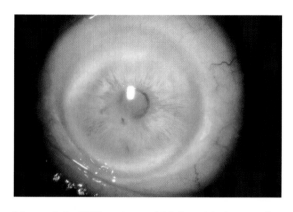

Figure 6.6 Diffuse interstitial keratitis in a patient with congenital syphilis. Slit lamp examination reveals ghost vessels deep in the stroma close to Descemet's membrane

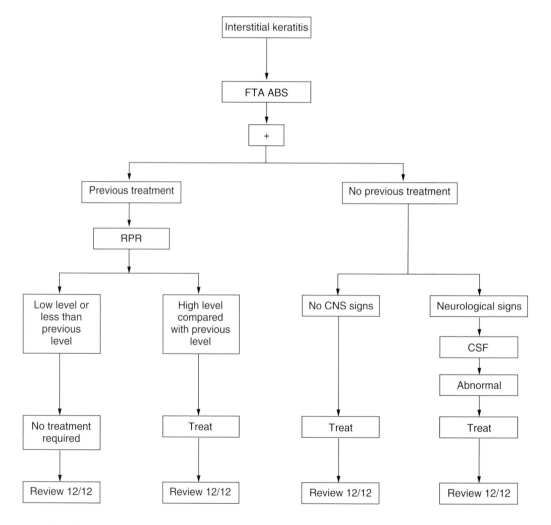

Figure 6.7 Antitreponemal treatment for patients with syphilitic interstitial keratitis

Syphilitic interstitial keratitis

Interstitial keratitis can be part of congenital syphilis or may complicate acquired secondary or tertiary disease.

Stromal inflammation may occur early in patients with congenital syphilis or years later and may recur through to middle life; it is bilateral and diffuse in distribution or, less commonly, multifocal. Neovascularisation is common and the vessels tend to be deep down, close to Descemet's membrane. When the inflammation resolves, ghost vessels remain and persist indefinitely (Figure 6.6).

Patients with interstitial keratitis due to congenital syphilis often have other characteristic features, such as malformed teeth, deafness, saddle nose deformity, and abnormalities of the skin.

Acquired disease is less common, tends to be multifocal rather than diffuse, and is often unilateral, and neovascularisation is less common than with the congenital form.

If syphilis is suspected, serological testing is mandatory; FTA-abs is the appropriate test. If positive and there are signs of neurosyphilis, a lumbar puncture for CSF studies should be considered. The requirements for diagnosing and treating patients with syphilis are set out in Figure 6.7.

Topical corticosteroids are the treatment of choice. The role of penicillin treatment for stromal keratitis remains controversial and should be considered in consultation with an appropriate physician.

Cogan's syndrome

Interstitial keratitis resembling that seen with congenital syphilis is often associated with

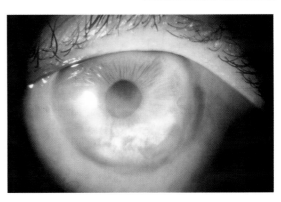

Figure 6.8 Cogan's syndrome. Interstitial keratitis with contiguous scleritis and nerve deafness resembling the pattern of disease found in syphilitic keratitis but with negative syphilis serology

contiguous scleritis and nerve deafness, but with negative syphilis serology is referred to as Cogan's syndrome (Figure 6.8). The cause is unknown. Treatment of this rare syndrome is limited to the use of topical corticosteroids.

Further reading

Baum J, Barza M, Weinstein P *et al*. Bilateral keratitis as a manifestation of Lyme disease. *Ophthalmology* 1988; **105**: 75.

Cobo LM, Foulks GN, Liesegang T *et al*. Oral acyclovir in the treatment of acute herpes zoster ophthalmicus. *Ophthalmology* 1986; **93**: 763.

Cogan DG. Syndrome of nonsyphilitic interstitial keratitis and vestibuloauditory symptoms. *Arch Ophthalmology* 1945; **33**: 144.

Matoba AY, Wilhelmus KR, Jones DB. Epstein–Barr viral stromal keratitis. *Ophthalmology* 1986; **93**: 746.

Orlin SE, Lauffer JL. Lyme disease keratitis (letter). *Am J Ophthalmology* 1989; **107**: 678.

Strauss SE, Cohen JI, Tosato G *et al*. Epstein–Barr virus: biology, pathogenesis and management. *Ann Intern Med* 1993; **118**: 45.

Tamesis RR, Foster S. Ocular syphilis. *Ophthalmology* 1990; **97**: 1281.

Wilhelmus KR. Ocular involvement in infectious mononucleosis. *Am J Ophthalmology* 1981; **91**: 117.

7 Proliferative lesions

Lumps and bumps on the surface of the cornea can arise from a range of pathological processes. Organ dysgenesis is responsible for dermoid development and, at the other end of the pathological scale, degenerative processes result in the creation of pinguecula and pterygia. Pseudopterygia, on the other hand, are a result of chronic inflammation. Neoplasia is uncommon in the cornea; when it occurs, it is confined to the epithelium with both benign papillomata and invasive carcinomata occurring.

Limbal dermoid

Dermoids are present at birth and are the result of disorganised development in the ocular region. They are often accompanied by evidence of a developmental aberration extending beyond the cornea in the presence of lid defects. Sometimes the developmental abnormality involves the face extensively (Figure 7.1).

Dermoids vary in size. They may be so small as to be insignificant or so large as to occlude all vision. They occur at the limbus, usually at the lower temporal quadrant, and are elevated lesions with evidence of skin and skin appendages in them. Usually they are superficial and involve the superficial stroma, but can occasionally be deeper.

Not all dermoids need to be treated. Cosmesis is the usual indication, but surgery is best left until the patient is a young adult and able to take some responsibility for the decision making. Sometimes it is necessary for the treatment to be carried out in childhood.

Treatment for visual defects associated with a dermoid is not nearly so successful and should be avoided wherever possible. Dermoids are almost invariably unilateral and even when successfully removed, it is very difficult to provide the retina with the quality of image that is necessary to match the other eye and to avoid amblyopia. Visual results are therefore poor.

When treatment is required, the procedure entails resection of the lesion and repair of the defect with a corneoscleral allograft. A trephine is used to mark the host cornea beyond the lesion. Then a lamella dissection is performed beneath the lesion and extending out into the sclera. An identical piece of donor cornea and sclera is then dissected from a whole globe and the corneal edge is inlaid into the corneal defect. The scleral edge is then sewn in. The repair of

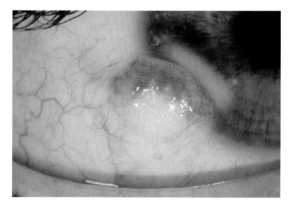

Figure 7.1 Limbal dermoid. A development lesion usually found at the lower temporal limbus, sometimes associated with a lid defect

the scleral edge does not require the same level of anatomical precision as the corneal edge which must be closed as accurately as possible. Closure is completed by sewing the conjunctival edge to the limbus, covering the scleral position of the graft.

Pterygium

Pterygia are fleshy lesions which occur at the corneal limbus, usually the nasal limbus, on the horizontal axis (Figure 7.2). Occasionally they occur at the corresponding position on the temporal limbus. Pterygia occurring elsewhere on the limbus should be suspected of being something else.

The pathological changes in these lesions include degeneration of elastin and collagen and fibrosis. These changes occur in patients who have been exposed to high levels of ultraviolet radiation, particularly in dry, dusty environments. Theories have been advanced to explain the nasal preponderance of pterygia on the basis of the focusing of ambient ultraviolet light at the medial limbus.

Patients with pterygia may be troubled by recurrent inflammation, the appearance of the lesion or, less commonly, visual disturbance. Inflammation is a consequence of the irregular corneal surface produced by the pterygium which disturbs the tear film and, in turn, compromises the nutrition of the corneal epithelium.

Visual disturbance can result from occlusion of the optical zone of the cornea or from astigmatism if the fibrosis in the pterygium contracts to flatten the cornea in the horizontal meridian.

Treatment is not always necessary and should be discouraged without a compelling indication. Loss of vision is such an indication. Recurrent inflammation and unhappiness with the appearance of the lesion are more relative indications.

Treatment, when indicated, is surgical, although some relief from bouts of inflammation can be gained from the use of lubricants and anti-inflammatory agents. There is, however, some debate as to the preferred surgical procedure.

Excision is often complicated by recurrence and recurrences are often more troublesome than the primary lesion. β Irradiation was used for many years but was complicated by scleral and corneal necrosis many years after surgery. This is a serious complication of irradiation which can result in loss of the eye in severe cases. For this reason the use of adjunctive radiotherapy has been abandoned in most places.

More recently, the use of cytotoxic agents has been advocated as an adjunct to surgery, but there have been some unsatisfactory complications reported, even in the short term.

Another adjunct to excisional surgery has been the use of various forms of flap repair. Pedicled and free grafts of conjunctiva and limbus have yielded excellent results, although the rates of cure have not been as great as reported for excision and β irradiation.

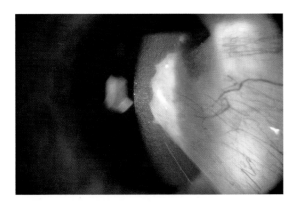

Figure 7.2 Pterygium, a proliferation of limbal tissue, usually at the medial limbus, caused by adverse environmental conditions, particularly excessive UV exposure

Pinguecula

Pinguecula are degenerative lesions in the conjunctiva occurring in similar localities as pterygia. Lipid accumulation is a feature and they have a characteristic yellow appearance. Some consider them to be the precursors of

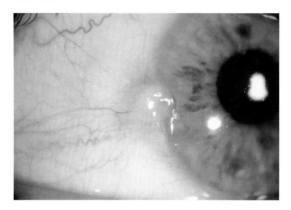

Figure 7.3 Pingueculum. A degenerative lesion in the conjunctival limbus

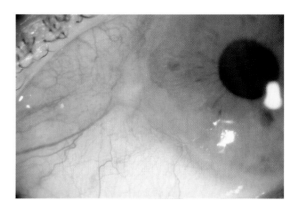

Figure 7.4 Corneal intraepithelial carcinoma. The abnormal epithelium is thicker and more opaque than normal corneal epithelium and a vasculature develops in the thickened limbal areas

pterygia, but not all progress to that. If unsightly, simple excision is appropriate and effective (Figure 7.3).

Intraepithelial neoplasia and squamous carcinoma

Conjunctival or corneal intraepithelial neoplasia (CIN) is a term used to describe dysplasia and neoplasia occurring in, and confined to, the epithelium of the cornea or conjunctiva. This classification has simplified the consideration of a group of conditions known in the past by such terms as Bowen's disease, intraepithelioma, intraepithelial intraepithelioma, intraepithelial carcinoma, carcinoma *in situ*, and intraepithelial dysplasia.

There is a progression from dysplasia to intraepithelial neoplasia and invasive carcinoma. Not all cases complete the progression but when this does occur, all three types of change may be seen on the one specimen.

Intraepithelial dysplasia and intraepithelial neoplasia of the cornea appear as areas of opacity in the epithelium indistinguishable from each other on clinical grounds. In the conjunctiva, the appearance may be different. The epithelium becomes thicker and a blood supply is required. The vessels grow up into the thickened conjunctiva and have the shape of a fir tree, with a central trunk growing towards the surface and smaller lateral branches (Figure 7.4).

Squamous carcinoma has a different appearance, with a gelatinous thickening of the conjunctiva or cornea and an arrangement of new vessels. The ingrowth of the vessels comes from conjunctival, episcleral, and scleral vessels which dilate to provide additional blood supply. These vessels can become large and obvious and are described as sentinel vessels (Figure 7.5).

The clinical course is slow and predictable. Metastases are uncommon, although local extension in extreme cases can be difficult to manage.

The histological appearance of the lesion is also predictable. The process arises in the depths of the limbal epithelium, perhaps in the limbal

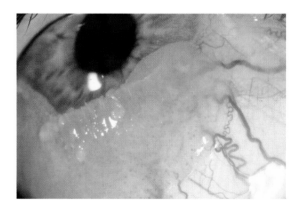

Figure 7.5 Squamous carcinoma of the cornea. The abnormal tissue is usually thick and opaque with large feeding vessels

stem cells. The abnormal cells move centrally and towards the surface as the process becomes more extensive. Dysplastic epithelial cells are usually elongated spindle cells with a high degree of similarity and regularity. Transformation can occur and at first these changes are confined to the epithelium. When the process breaks through the basement membrane, the diagnosis becomes invasive squamous carcinoma (Figure 7.6).

The cause of the dysplastic and neoplastic processes is unclear. The disease is much more common in men than women and is more common in warm sunny environments, but is curiously unilateral. This suggests that at least two factors are necessary for the process, one being ultraviolet light and the other as yet unknown, although papilloma virus has been suggested as the second agent.

Excision is the established treatment. The use of adjunctive cryotherapy is also advocated because of the high recurrence rates with excision alone. When excising these lesions, attention must be paid to removing the limbus from which the process is arising. This should be done with sharp dissection to remove the deep nest of aberrant stem cells. The area of abnormal limbus should be completely excised. The corneal epithelium can be debrided with a blunt knife or scalpel. It is not necessary to remove any stroma unless there has been previous surgery which makes

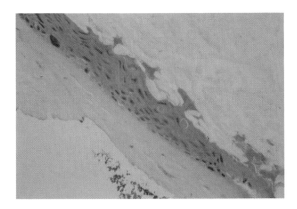

Figure 7.6 Squamous cell carcinoma of the cornea. Histological section showing neoplastic cells breaching the epithelial basement membrane

delineation of the recurrent epithelial lesion difficult.

Even when the lesion is completely excised, recurrence is common, not necessarily arising from the previously excised lesion. It is as though the entire limbus is at risk of developing the pathological change once the process has affected one part of the eye. Recurrences often appear away from previous lesions in areas of limbus that were previously normal.

When planning therapy, the field change phenomena must be taken into account. Recurrences are likely to occur in other areas of the limbus and the lesion and the treatment are likely to compromise more of the limbus. If this occurs a number of times or if recurrence is extensive, limbal failure may occur and vision be compromised. Excisions should be precise, preserving as much of the limbus as possible but completely removing the lesion. The completeness of the excision must be checked with the pathologist and, if incomplete, further excision can be carried out but may compromise the result.

This raises questions about the advisability of cryotherapy. A double freeze-thaw, using an appropriately designed cryoprobe, reduces recurrences when compared to excision alone, but the technique is relatively imprecise and there is no assessment of its long term effect. There is widespread injury to the limbus which can be complicated by limbal insufficiency and widespread epithelial disturbance. A case can thus be made for excision alone. However, the accepted treatment at present is excision and cryotherapy.

Recently, the use of topical mitomycin C has been advocated. Encouraging results are common but this approach remains in a developmental phase.

Papillomata

Papillomata of the conjunctiva and cornea are common, benign lesions which can occur anywhere on the conjunctiva and which sometimes occur at the limbus. They grow

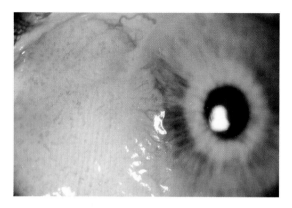

Figure 7.7 Benign papillomata of the corneal limbus. The lesion is gelatinous with an obvious circulation. There is no tendency to involve the central corneal epithelium

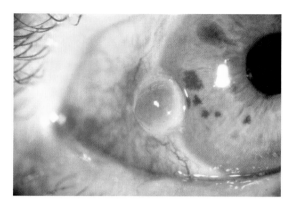

Figure 7.8 Granuloma of the conjunctiva and limbus – an excessive growth of granulation tissue which occurs in the vicinity of a healing wound

quickly and usually present because the patient becomes alarmed by their appearance (Figure 7.7).

The lesions vary in size from barely perceptible to large. They have a red, gelatinous appearance due to the proliferation of blood vessels in the mass of epithelial cells and are often friable and bleed. Sometimes they secrete mucus.

Histological examination reveals a mass of proliferating epithelial cells with supporting interstitium and vasculature. There is no evidence of malignant transformation. Infection with papilloma virus is the cause, although this cannot be proved in every case.

Treatment is excisional biopsy.

Granuloma of the conjunctiva and limbus

Occasionally, after a break in the conjunctiva or limbus due to trauma or surgery, an exuberant and excessive growth of granulation tissue occurs in the vicinity of the healing wound (Figure 7.8). The lesion appears as an inflamed and infected lump on the surface of the eye. Histological examination reveals a mass of granulation tissue. Patients are concerned by the appearance of the lump which may bleed and discharge a little purulent material.

The natural history of the condition is spontaneous resolution but this may take an unacceptable time, perhaps weeks or sometimes months. Topical corticosteroids are usually effective in bringing about resolution in a few days. In recalcitrant cases, excision and topical steroids are likely to be curative.

Further reading

Ash JE, Wilder HC. Epithelial tumors of the limbus. *Am J Ophthalmol* 1942; **25**: 926.
Boockvar W, Wessely Z, Ballen P. Recurrent granuloma pyogenicum of limbus. *Arch Ophthalmol* 1974; **91**: 42.
Dailey EG, Lubowitz RM. Dermoids of the limbus and cornea. *Am J Ophthalmol* 1962; **53**: 661.
Elsas FJ, Green WR. Epibulbar tumors in childhood. *Am J Ophthalmol* 1975; **79**: 1001.
Erie JC, Campbell RJ, Liesegang TJ. Conjunctival and corneal intraepithelial and invasive neoplasia. *Ophthalmology* 1986; **93**: 176.
Kenyon KR, Wagoner MD, Hettinger ME. Conjunctival autograft transplantation for advanced and recurrent pterygium. *Ophthalmology* 1985; **92**: 1461.
Mackenzie FD, Hirst LW, Battistutta D, Gren A. Risk analysis in the development of pterygia. *Ophthalmology* 1992; **99**: 1056.
Mackenzie FD, Hirst LW, Kynaston B, Bain C. Recurrence rate and complications after beta irradiation for pterygia. *Ophthalmology* 1991; **98**: 1776.
Starck T, Kenyon KR, Serrano F. Conjunctival autograft for primary and recurrent pterygia: surgical technique and problem management. *Cornea* 1991; **10**: 196.

8 Corneal ectasia: acquired abnormalities of corneal shape

Conditions in which the cornea becomes thin and loses tensile strength, and subsequently develops warpage and irregular astigmatism, are referred to as corneal ectasias. The maintenance of a corneal shape appropriate to focus a precise image on the retina is essential for good vision and ectatic conditions of the cornea can cause very poor vision.

Acquired abnormalities of corneal shape are common, can be very damaging to vision and difficult to manage. Four conditions deserve discussion: keratoconus, keratoglobus, pellucid marginal degeneration, and Terrien's marginal degeneration. The first three may be the same condition but Terrien's is distinctly different. However, in all four conditions, thinning of the cornea, with a decrease in tensile strength, is the underlying abnormality accounting for the change in corneal shape. Of these conditions known collectively as corneal ectasias, keratoconus is the most important. The morphological differences between keratoconus, pellucid marginal degeneration, and keratoglobus are shown in Figure 8.1.

Keratoconus

Keratoconus is a common disorder, that is especially prevalent in Western communities at approximately 50–200 per 100 000 people. The incidence varies across racial groups. Although the condition is more common in some families, most cases are sporadic and no particular pattern of inheritance is apparent.

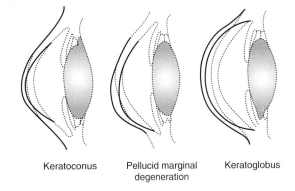

Keratoconus   Pellucid marginal degeneration   Keratoglobus

Figure 8.1 In keratoconus the area of maximal thinning is central and the contour conical. With pellucid marginal degeneration thinning is maximal inferiorly, as is the curvature; the central cornea may be quite flat. In keratoglobus the cornea is large and thin and the contour bulbous

Keratoconus has various forms of clinical expression. The essential shared features are corneal thinning and irregular astigmatism. Ectasia is a term used to describe not only thinning but weakening of the cornea. This may result from abnormalities of the collagen, changes within the ground substance, or a decreased thickness of normal stroma.

Ocular and systemic associations

For the most part, keratoconus occurs as an isolated ocular finding. It can, however, be found in association with other disorders. The most commonly encountered association is with atopy, although the reason is yet to be determined. It is an association of some significance as these patients tend to be young, intolerant of contact lenses, and tend to develop more inflammatory complications after surgery. Neither is the well known association with Leber's amourosis explainable. Keratoconus is also associated with Down's syndrome and a number of conditions with abnormalities of connective tissue, including Ehlers–Danlos syndrome, Marfan's syndrome, and mitral valve prolapse.

Clinical features

Keratoconus usually manifests in the first three decades of life. Its effect is to impair vision. Myopia is usually the first manifestation and as the condition progresses, irregular astigmatism develops, making spectacle correction of the myopia unsatisfactory. Hard contact lenses provide better quality of vision.

The most obvious clinical signs are of irregular myopic astigmatism. This may be first apparent from the retinoscopy, the subjective refraction, or keratometry. Decreased corneal thickness and increased corneal curvature may be apparent from the slit lamp examination but are not usually apparent in mild cases. However, even a mild increase in corneal curvature can facilitate specular reflection of Descemet's membrane and the corneal endothelium, making their visualisation much more obvious. In some cases, the conical shape of the cornea is so obvious that it can be seen with the naked eye. The cone is easier to see if the clinician looks down across the patient's brow to see the cone protruding from behind the upper lid. This is described as *Munson's sign*.

Box 8.1 *Systemic conditions associated with keratoconus*

Down's syndrome
Leber's congenital amourosis
Atopic disease
Ehlers–Danlos syndrome
Marfan's syndrome
Mitral valve prolapse
Floppy eyelid syndrome

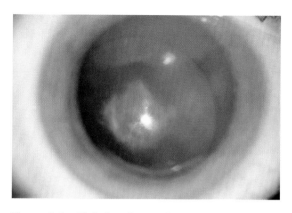

Figure 8.2 Fleischer line, a line of iron deposition around the base of a cone

Other slit lamp signs include an iron line around the base of the cone, particularly inferiorly, known as a *Fleischer line* (Figure 8.2). This deposition of iron is at the level of Bowman's membrane and has an appearance very similar to a Hudson–Stahle line.

There may also be a series of vertical, white parallel lines at the level of Bowman's membrane at the apex of the cone. These are called *Vogt's striae*.

In severe cases, splits or ruptures in Descemet's membrane may occur. If large, they will allow fluid into the stroma, creating an opaque area which can be so extensive as to involve the whole cornea. This condition, known as *corneal hydrops* (Figure 8.3), usually resolves

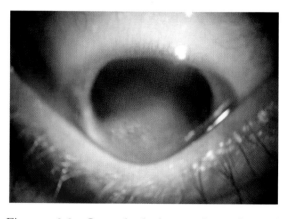

Figure 8.3 Corneal hydrops. In advanced keratoconus slits may develop in Descemet's membrane, causing a break in the endothelium and focal corneal oedema

and vision returns to its level before the rupture or may be improved if the healing process has scarred the cornea into a less curved shape. The site of the rupture, however, is always apparent.

There may also be scarring in the more superficial layers of the cornea. This tends to be in the vicinity of the apex of the cone and occurs immediately under the epithelium. Apical scarring can be marked in patients who have been wearing contact lenses that are too flat and rest on the apex of the cone.

Keratoconus is almost invariably bilateral but seldom symmetrical. In cases appearing to be unilateral, a close look at the other eye will almost always reveal some evidence of the disease. This may be as minimal as a slightly irregular retinoscopy reflex or a mildly abnormal corneal topography plot. The subclinical form of the disease has traditionally been called *keratoconus forme fruste*.

Confirmation of the clinical diagnosis rests on acquiring quantitative data. Accurate measurement of the corneal curvature and corneal thickness is required. Corneal curvature can be measured by keratometry, an approach used for many years. The limitation of keratometry is that it provides information about the central optical zone only. Although this is the critical area of the cornea as far as corneal refraction of light is concerned, there can be a lot going on in the cornea outside the optical zone in keratoconus. Changes in the peripheral cornea may be relevant to interpreting the whole clinical picture or arranging therapeutic interventions, such as contact lens fitting or surgery. For this reason, corneal topography is now widely used to plot the anterior curvature of the cornea in patients with keratoconus (Figure 8.4). This approach also emphasises the recurring patterns of morphological change occurring in the corneas of these patients. Increased central corneal curvature, a greater than usual difference between the central and peripheral corneal curvature, and a flatter curve in the superior cornea than inferiorly are topographical features characteristic of keratoconus (Figure 8.5).

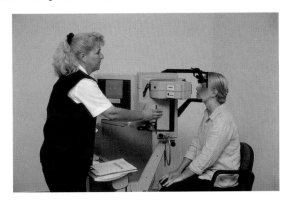

Figure 8.4 Videokeratography has become a common clinical investigation

Corneal thickness can be measured optically or with ultrasound and some topography packages provide corneal thickness measurements as well as data about curvature. What is particularly important is assessment of the thickness of the cornea over its entire extent if surgery is being considered. An area of marked peripheral thinning needs to be considered if surgery is planned.

Treatment

The optimal approach to the treatment of keratoconus can be summarised as follows: patients should be encouraged to wear spectacles in the first instance, until they become ineffective or unacceptable to the patient. They should then be managed with semi-rigid gas permeable contact lenses. Surgery, in the form of penetrating corneal transplantation, should only be considered if the contact lens option fails.

Contact lens failure can be defined as the inability to wear contact lenses prescribed and supervised by someone experienced in fitting contact lenses to patients with keratoconus. The overwhelming majority of patients with keratoconus can be managed with contact lenses. Only 1–2% of patients with keratoconus will ever require surgery. However the patient is managed, there is need for long term encouragement and support. It is important for the clinician to provide not only the technical support but personal encouragement to patients

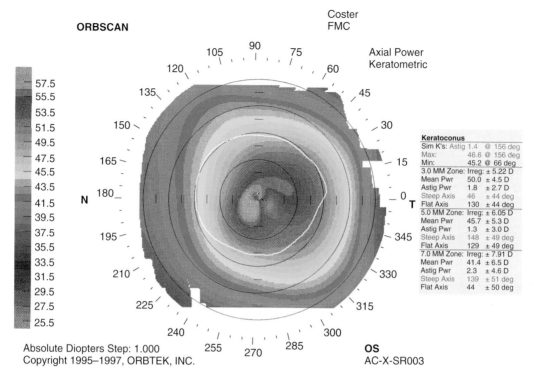

Figure 8.5 Keratoconus. Topography demonstrates increased central corneal curvature, greater than normal difference between central and peripheral corneal curvature, with the inferior corneal curvature steeper than the superior cornea

so that they can cope with an affliction which is a lifelong disorder. Although the need for support cannot be overlooked, it is also important to emphasise to patients with keratoconus that one way or another and given average luck, they will be able to live a normal life unencumbered by visual disability. Those who require surgery have an approximately 90% chance of achieving, and maintaining, 6/12 vision.

Contact lens fitting

In all but the simplest cases, because keratoconus represents a significant challenge to the contact lens practitioner, it is preferable to have this aspect managed by someone with relevant experience. Fitting contact lenses to patients with keratoconus has been compared to fitting shoes to someone with clubfeet. Essentially, it is an art based on trial and error, but there are some guiding principles.

First, a rigid or semi-rigid material is always preferable to a soft lens, even though this may not be quite as comfortable, at least initially. Second, the lens should ride on the periphery of the cornea; this usually demands that a lens with more than one posterior surface curve be used. Third, there should be apical clearance so that there is a minimal chance of creating apical scarring.

Since there is considerable variability in the extent and severity of the corneal changes in keratoconus, some fittings can be extremely difficult. The importance of achieving a contact lens fit rather than resorting to corneal transplantation should spur the clinician on to do whatever is required.

In the event of contact lens failure, surgery is indicated. Contact lens failure may occur because the cornea is too misshapen to fit or because the eye is too sensitive to tolerate a lens. Alternatively, the patient may develop a complication of lens wear, such as giant capillary conjunctivitis. If the cornea is too misshapen to fit, surgery may be considered. All the other difficulties can be seen as relative contraindications.

Some patients are averse to the idea of contact lens wear, but this is not a good reason for considering surgery instead. In these patients, it is appropriate to attempt to change their attitude to lens wear because it is in their best long term interest. Even if they are suited to corneal transplantation, they may still need a contact lens postoperatively to achieve their full visual potential.

Surgery for keratoconus

Penetrating corneal transplantation is the procedure of choice for patients with keratoconus who are no longer manageable with contact lenses. Other procedures, such as thermokeratoplasty, epikeratoplasty, and lamellar transplantation, have been advocated at different times but none have stood the test of time. The best published visual results come from penetrating corneal transplantation.

Keratoconus is the most common indication for corneal transplantation in most Western countries. In excess of 90% of patients receiving corneal transplants for keratoconus achieve 6/12 or better, although it may take several years to reach this level of vision. Some patients do not do quite as well as others. There is a strong link between atopy and keratoconus and this group of patients is more likely to develop inflammation postoperatively. This predisposes them to suture loosening and allograft rejection. Patients with eccentric cones that need eccentric grafts are also prone to rejection. Similarly, patients with excessive peripheral corneal thinning are prone to wound complications and astigmatism.

Management of penetrating transplantation for keratoconus

At the time of surgery it is necessary to decide on the size and position of the graft and the suture pattern. The size should be that which allows for maximum graft survival and large enough to encompass the cone and allow for some expansion of the cone with passing years. This usually means a graft of 7.5–8.5 mm. If the cone is eccentric, it is usually necessary to compromise with regard to placement of the graft, centring it between the centre of the cone and the visual axis.

The suture pattern is not critical in that no one pattern has been shown to reduce astigmatism, although many have been advocated. One preference is for a continuous 10/0 nylon suture (Figure 8.6). This technique is simple and quick and creates no more astigmatism than any other technique. In young patients with atopy, however, interrupted sutures are preferred because of the propensity of these patients to develop inflammation around sutures, causing suture loosening. This is easier to manage with interrupted sutures because individual sutures can be removed without compromising the wound.

Postoperatively, topical corticosteroids are used to suppress inflammation, thereby reducing the possibility of allograft rejection. Prednisolone phosphate eye drops are used four times a day for the first six months and then reduced to three times a day for the next three months.

At 12 months, suture removal is considered. If there are less than five dioptres of astigmatism and the patient sees well, the sutures are left in

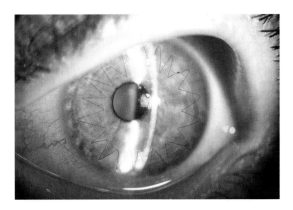

Figure 8.6 Corneal transplant for keratoconus secured with a continuous 10.0 nylon suture

97

for another three or six months in the expectation that the acceptable corneal shape will become more stable with time. If, however, there are more than five dioptres of astigmatism and the patient sees badly, it is as well to remove the suture at 12 months and proceed with whatever is required to achieve the best possible visual result. This involves refraction and the provision of spectacles or contact lenses and may involve incisional surgery to reduce regular astigmatism.

Postoperative astigmatism is a problem in all groups of patients receiving corneal transplants but is particularly troublesome in patients with keratoconus. This is because the peripheral host cornea is usually of irregular thickness and strength and the support of the optical zone of the cornea is irregular, resulting in warpage. Such irregularities can also make cutting and suturing more difficult, further contributing to astigmatism. Most of the astigmatism found after corneal transplantation is manageable with optical aids or simple incisional surgery. The average amount of corneal astigmatism after penetrating corneal transplantation for keratoconus is around 4 dioptres, measured by keratometry.

Astigmatism can develop decades after successful corneal transplantation. This occurs because the ectatic process continues to progress after surgery. It may be confined to the central cornea initially, but over decades progresses to involve the whole cornea so that the host cornea outside the graft thins and the wound in the vicinity of the thinning stretches to produce flattening in that meridian.

Keratoglobus

It is reasonable to consider keratoglobus as an extreme form of keratoconus in which all of the cornea is involved, with the extrusion of the cornea being bulbous rather than conical (Figure 8.7). Keratoglobus is more often associated with systemic connective tissue disorders than is the case in patients with a conical cornea. The principles of management are the

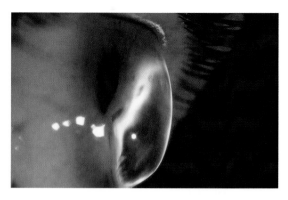

Figure 8.7 Keratoglobus. The cornea is large, thin, and bulbous in profile with the central cornea flat rather than steep. Commonly keratoglobus is part of a systemic connective tissue disorder

same as for other less striking forms of the disease but the extreme shape of the cornea and thinness provide serious challenges for the contact lens fitter and surgeon.

Pellucid marginal degeneration

This condition is also best thought of as a variant of keratoconus. It is reasonable to think of it as a condition in which the ectatic process responsible for keratoconus in some patients affects the periphery of the cornea (Figure 8.8). There is thinning of the peripheral cornea, usually inferiorly, so that the curvature is maximal in the periphery. The central cornea may be quite flat (Figure 8.9). Again the

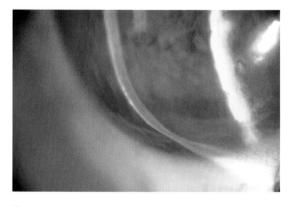

Figure 8.8 Pellucid marginal degeneration. Thinning occurs in the peripheral inferior cornea. Corneal curvature is greatest in the inferior peripheral cornea and the central cornea may be flat

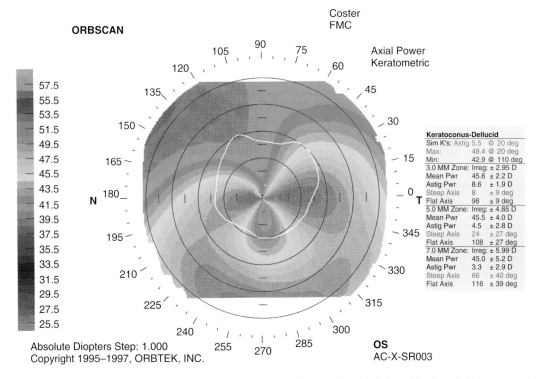

Figure 8.9 Pellucid marginal degeneration. Videokeratography confirms inferior thinning, inferior steepening, and flat superior cornea

principles of management are the same as for other expressions of keratoconus, but the practicalities can be difficult. Contact lens fitting to such an abnormally shaped cornea is challenging. Surgery is also difficult because the host cornea is very thin in the area of the inferior wound margin. Sometimes the anticipated difficulties in conventional penetrating corneal transplantation are such that alternatives are necessary. Resection of the thin peripheral cornea and direct suture has been used and so too have peripheral onlay corneal lamellar grafts.

Terrien's marginal dystrophy

This rare condition is obviously different from the keratoconus variants described above. However, there is a shared feature in that Terrien's dystrophy produces irregular corneal astigmatism. This arises because of an atrophic process that weakens the support given by the peripheral cornea to the central optical zone.

The clinical features of the disease include onset of visual loss as a consequence of unstable astigmatism. The condition usually appears in mid-life. The peripheral cornea is thin and atrophic with vascularisation and lipid deposition (Figure 8.10). This process may occur more in some areas of the peripheral

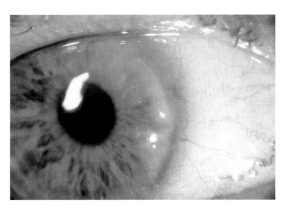

Figure 8.10 Terrien's dystrophy. The peripheral cornea is atrophic with vascularisation and lipid deposition

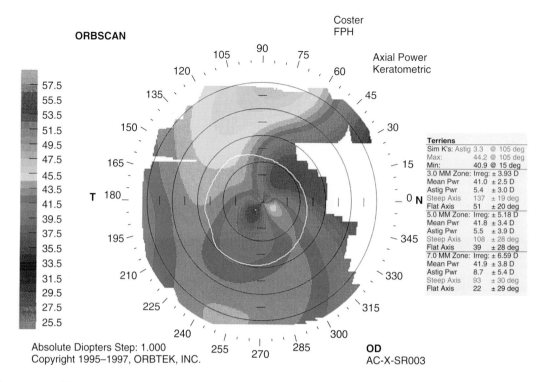

Figure 8.11 Terrien's dystrophy. There is thinning and distortion of the peripheral cornea with central irregular astigmatism

cornea than in others. Refraction reveals an astigmatic cornea which can be confirmed with topography (Figure 8.11). Usually both eyes are affected but not symmetrically.

There is seldom much inflammation and, in the majority of cases, the eyes are not clinically inflamed, although there may be a suggestion of inflammation on slit lamp examination. Occasionally there is obvious inflammation. This suggests that in some cases the condition may be a mild form of the destructive process underlying Mooren's ulceration, a condition in which there is peripheral corneal destruction with ulceration and a marked inflammatory response. Perhaps the two conditions are opposite ends of a spectrum.

Treatment is challenging. The natural history of the condition is to persist with unresolving astigmatism and this may be of sufficient order as to demand treatment in bilateral cases. Contact lens fitting is the most satisfactory approach but

this is not an option in the most severe cases where there may be as much as 30 dioptres of astigmatism. In these cases, surgery must be considered. The most satisfactory surgical alternative is a peripheral onlay corneal graft.

Age-related peripheral corneal atrophy

This condition resembles Terrien's dystrophy in that there is thinning of the peripheral cornea with a tendency to vascularisation and lipid deposition. As the name implies, the condition comes on late in life. The features resemble Terrien's dystrophy but are not as marked and astigmatism is not a problem. Perhaps the two conditions are also opposite ends of a spectrum. Treatment is not required.

Further reading

Baum J. On the location of the cone and the etiology of keratoconus. *Cornea* 1995; **14**: 142–3.

Bron AJ. Keratoconus. *Cornea* 1988; 7: 163.

Copeman PWM. Eczema and keratoconus. *BMJ* 1965; **2**: 977.

Etzine S. Conical cornea in identical twins. *South Afr Med J* 1954; **28**: 154–5.

Etzine S, Friedmann A. Marginal dystrophy of the cornea with total ectasia. *Am J Ophthalmol* 1963; **55**: 150.

Gasset AR, Kaufman HE. Thermokeratoplasty in the treatment of keratoconus. *Am J Ophthalmol* 1975; **79**: 226–32.

Halliday BL. Epikeratophakia for aphakia, keratoconus, and myopia. *Br J Ophthalmol* 1990; **74**: 67–72.

Hanson IM, Fletcher JM, Jordan T *et al*. Mutations at the PAX 6 locus are found in heterogeneous anterior segment malformations including Peters' anomaly. *Nat Genet* 1994; **6**: 168–73.

Harrison RJ, Klouda PT, Easty DL *et al*. Association of keratoconus and atopy. *Br J Ophthalmol* 1989; **73**: 816.

Jacobs HB. Posterior conical cornea. *Br J Ophthalmol* 1957; **41**: 31.

Jefferies LW, Alexander RA. Connective tissue fibre production in keratoconus. *Br J Biomed Sci* 1995; **52**: 14–18.

Krachmer HH, Feder RS, Belin MW. Keratoconus and related non-inflammatory corneal thinning disorders. *Surv Ophthalmol* 1984; **28**: 293–322.

Krachmer J. Pellucid marginal corneal degeneration. *Arch Ophthalmol* 1978; **96**: 1217.

Lowe RF. The eyes in mongolism. *Br J Ophthalmol* 1949; **33**: 131.

Maguire LJ, Lowry J. Identifying progression of subclinical keratoconus by serial topography analysis. *Am J Ophthalmol* 1991; **112**: 41.

Mannis MJ. Iron deposition in the corneal graft. *Arch Ophthalmol* 1983; **101**: 1858.

Meire FM, Bleeker-Wagemakers EM, Oheler M *et al*. X-linked megalocornea. Ocular findings and linkage analysis. *Ophthalmic Paediatr Genet* 1991; **12**: 153–7.

Pearce WG. Autosomal dominant megalocornea with congenital glaucoma: evidence for germ-line mosaicism. *Can J Ophthalmol* 1991; **26**: 21–6.

Rabinowitz YS, McDonnell PJ. Computer-assisted corneal topography in keratoconus. *Refract Corneal Surg* 1989; **5**: 400–8.

Rabinowitz YS. Keratoconus. *Surv Ophthalmol* 1988; **42**: 297–319.

Rabinowitz YW. Videokeratography indices to aid in screening for keratoconus. *J Refract Surg* 1995; **11**: 371–9.

Smith VA, Hoh HB, Littleton L *et al*. Over-expression of gelatinase. A activity in keratoconus. *Eye* 1995; **9**: 429–33.

Suveges I, Levai G, Alberth B. Pathology of Terrien's disease. *Am J Ophthalmol* 1972; **74**: 1191.

Terrien F. Dystrophie marginale symmetrique des duex cornées. *Arch Ophthalmol (Paris)* 1900; **20**: 12.

Wood TO. Lamellar transplants in keratoconus. *Am J Ophthalmol* 1977; **83**: 543.

Zhou L, Sawaguchi S, Twining SS *et al*. Expression of degradative enzymes and protease inhibitors in corneas with keratoconus. *Invest Ophthalmol Vis Sci* 1998; **39**: 1117–24.

9 Herpes simplex virus keratitis

Herpes simplex virus (HSV) keratitis is one of the most common conditions affecting the cornea. Various distinct patterns of clinical expression occur. The clinical features of HSV infection vary from patient to patient and in one patient over a period of time. Usually, patients are infected in childhood and those who develop recurrent disease may be troubled in some way for the rest of their lives.

Because of the wide range of clinical eye disease due to HSV infection and the way in which various apparently dissimilar conditions are linked, it is necessary to consider an overview of herpetic infection of the cornea and external eye.

Clinical appearances are determined by the direct pathological effect of the virus, with an important contribution from the host response.

The host response differs over a lifetime with the changing reactivity of the immune response and exposure to the virus.

Most people come into contact with the HSV in the first decade of life. Often this is the result of contact between a mother with a cold sore on her lip and her child. If the inoculation is in the eye, a primary ocular infection can occur. This may never become recurrent or it may be the beginning of corneal pathology evolving over a lifetime and resulting in visual loss. The pathways to visual loss in patients with ocular HSV are shown in Figure 9.1.

Primary ocular herpes simplex virus infection: blepharoconjunctivitis

Herpes simplex virus infection usually takes the form of blepharoconjunctivitis (Figure 9.2).

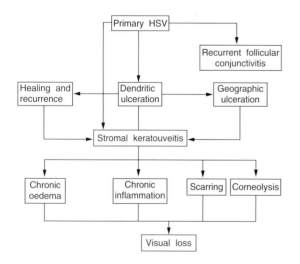

Figure 9.1   Pathways to visual loss from ocular herpes simplex virus infection

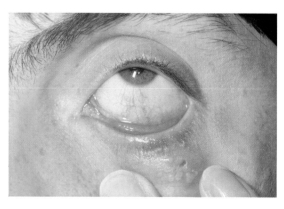

Figure 9.2   Primary ocular herpes simplex virus infection. Blepharoconjunctivitis with lid vesicles and follicular conjunctivitis

There are blisters on the lid margin and a follicular conjunctivitis. In addition, the cornea may be affected by punctate superficial keratitis (Figure 9.3) and even multiple small dendritic lesions. This picture can occur at any time in the first three or four decades of life.

Following primary infection, the virus travels up the sensory nerve to the trigeminal ganglion where it resides in a latent state, retaining the ability to become active at any time. When this happens, virus particles travel down the trigeminal nerves, are shed onto the mucosal surface and can then enter epithelial cells and create recurrent infection.

Dendritic keratitis

This is the most common form of recurrent HSV disease. The virus shed from the trigeminal nerve enters corneal epithelial cells where it replicates, creating a productive infection (Figure 9.4). The infected cells exhibit a direct cytopathic effect with the virus spreading from cell to cell in such a way as to create a branching pattern on the surface of the cornea. The affected cells stain readily with rose bengal. The most affected cells are shed from the surface of the cornea to reveal the underlying Bowman's membrane that stains with fluorescein. This is a true dendritic ulcer (Figure 9.5). Not all dendritic figures advance to the level of ulceration so the term dendritic keratitis is preferred to dendritic ulcer (Figure 9.6).

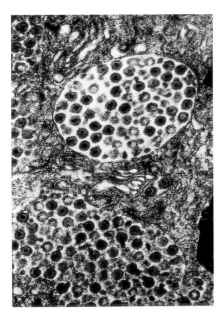

Figure 9.3 Primary ocular herpes simplex virus infection. Superficial punctate keratitis which is found in association with blepharokeratoconjunctivitis. The lesions are indistinguishable from the lesions caused by adenovirus and Chlamydia

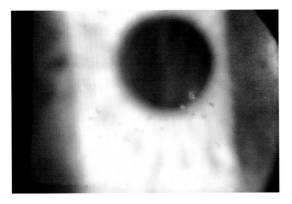

Figure 9.4 Herpes simplex virus infection of ocular surface epithelium. Electron micrograph to show cells stuffed with virus particles

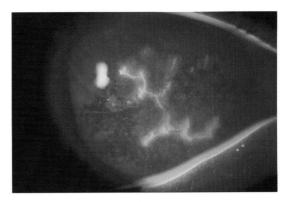

Figure 9.5 Dendritic ulceration of the cornea due to herpes simplex virus infection

Geographic ulceration

Geographic ulceration of the cornea occurs under circumstances that favour the spread of virus from cell to cell, usually due to the use of topical corticosteroids in someone who has HSV replicating in the cornea. Similarly,

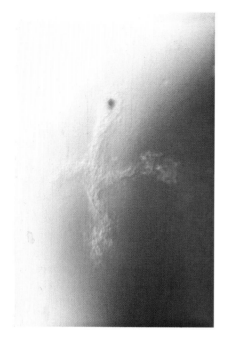

Figure 9.6 Dendritic figure in the corneal epithelium due to herpes simplex virus infection. The corneal foreign body was responsible for initiating the process

immunosuppression from medication or as part of systemic disease will also favour spread of virus from cell to cell, so that instead of the virus spreading along the cornea in a linear branching manner, it spreads rapidly from cell to cell in all directions. As infected cells are shed, large areas of Bowman's membrane are left denuded in geographic shapes (Figure 9.7). For purposes of

classification, an area of ulceration 0.5 mm across the lesion is described as a geographic ulcer. Originally, the term used was amoeboid ulcer but since the recognition in 1974 that amoebae can cause corneal ulceration, the term geographic ulcer has come to be preferred.

The infectious process may not be confined to the epithelium. The corneal stroma may also be involved. Important differences between epithelial and stromal infections with HSV reflect differences in the host response to viral antigens which create the clinical features of stromal disease. Virus replication and direct cytotoxicity are relatively less important in stromal disease than in epithelial disease where productive infection of epithelial cells is the principal pathological process.

Herpetic stromal keratitis

This occurs in two broad forms, irregular stromal keratitis and disciform stromal keratitis.

Irregular stromal keratitis

This is a condition in which there is patchy inflammatory change in the corneal stroma (Figure 9.8). This may occur as a complication of ulcerative herpetic disease or as a recurrent expression of the disease. Although viral antigens can be identified in the stroma, there is little

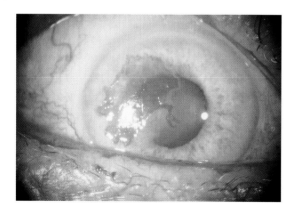

Figure 9.7 Geographic ulceration of the cornea due to herpes simplex virus infection

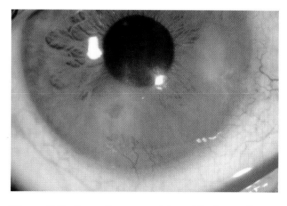

Figure 9.8 Irregular stromal keratitis due to herpes simplex virus infection. The inflammatory changes in the cornea are patchy (irregular). It can occur with or without corneal ulceration

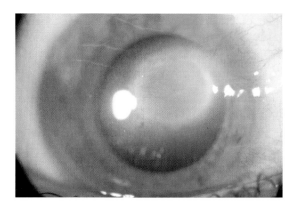

Figure 9.9 Disciform stromal keratitis due to herpes simplex virus. There is a disc of inflammatory oedema and cellular infiltrate in the corneal stroma. Usually the epithelium is intact

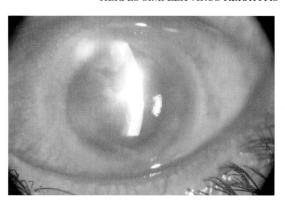

Figure 9.10 Metaherpetic corneal ulceration. Persistent inflammation in the base of the ulcer impairs epithelial healing

suspicion of viral replication being important in driving the process. There is, however, a prominent mononuclear cell infiltrate.

Disciform stromal keratitis

This is a condition which manifests clinically with a disc of inflammatory oedema and cellular infiltrate in the corneal stroma (Figure 9.9). This may occur as a complication of an overlying ulcer, but occurs more often when the corneal endothelium is intact. Viral antigen is detectable but virus replication is not thought to be important in driving the process. There may be infection of the endothelium of the cornea to account for the localised area of oedema. The disciform area of oedema may be central or eccentric.

Stromal inflammation is important in its own right but it may also affect the healing of corneal ulceration. Inflamed stroma is not an adequate substrate for the epithelium to heal over.

Metaherpetic ulceration

This term describes a corneal ulcer which will not heal because of the state of the underlying stroma. Such ulcers may occur when the virus is replicating in the corneal epithelium or after this phase has passed (Figure 9.10).

Herpetic uveitis

Herpetic uveitis is relatively common; the clinical signs are of an anterior uveitis, often with elevated intraocular pressure and with contiguous, non-segmental iris atrophy, and in many cases there is evidence of pre-existing or concurrent corneal inflammation (Figure 9.11).

Herpetic canaliculitis

Herpetic canaliculitis can occur as a complication of a primary infection of the conjunctival sac. The mid-canalicular portion of the lacrimal drainage system is affected and this

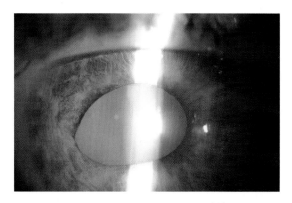

Figure 9.11 Herpetic uveitis. There is anterior uveitis, often with mildly elevated intraocular pressure, and irregular and scattered defects in the pigment epithelium of the iris. The iris defects transilluminate

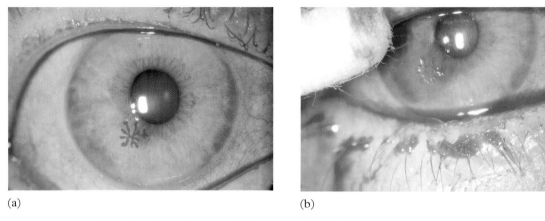

(a)   (b)

Figure 9.12   Dendritic keratitis before (a) and after (b) swab debridement

usually results in an obstruction that is difficult to deal with surgically.

Treatment of herpetic keratitis: the broad principles

The treatment of patients with herpetic eye disease is determined by the nature of the underlying pathology. Dendritic keratopathy and geographic ulceration are due to virus replication and are treated with antiviral agents which impair viral replication. Idoxuridine, acycloguanosine, and trifluorothymidine are available in preparations for topical use and are widely employed for this purpose. Delivered topically as drops or ointment, they are effective in treating epithelial conditions that are due to virus replication. They are even more effective if the virus load can be reduced, as it can in dendritic keratitis by mechanically removing infected cells by debriding them from the corneal surface with a cotton bud or similar implement (Figure 9.12). The treatment of stromal disease is more complicated, perhaps because the pathology of the condition is not so well understood.

The treatment of corneal stromal disease due to HSV infection aims at suppressing the damaging stromal inflammation. This is effectively done with topical corticosteroids, but at some risk. Amongst other things, topical steroids enhance viral replication in the epithelium. In order to negate this effect, topical steroids are administered to patients with herpetic keratitis in conjunction with antivirals to reduce the chance of encouraging subclinical infection or enhancing coexisting infection. As long as topical corticosteroids are used to treat herpetic stromal keratitis, it is necessary to administer topical antiviral to prevent the development of dendritic geographic ulceration. As it is usually necessary to treat herpetic keratitis with topical steroids over a prolonged period, usually about three months but often longer, it is necessary to use antivirals for most of this time. As a rule of thumb, the topical antiviral is maintained until the dose of topical steroids is reduced to as little as the equivalent of one drop a day of prednisolone phosphate 0.5%. The dose of prednisolone required is determined by the response to therapy; a usual starting point is prednisolone phosphate 0.5% four times a day. At each visit, the inflammatory reaction in the cornea is evaluated and the dose of prednisolone is regulated accordingly. In other words, the anti-inflammatory medication is titrated against the inflammatory reaction.

Further reading

Anonymous. A controlled trial of oral acyclovir for the prevention of stromal keratitis or iritis in patients with herpes simplex virus epithelial keratitis. *Arch Ophthalmol* 1997; **115**: 703–12.

Anonymous. Acyclovir for the prevention of recurrent herpes simplex virus eye disease. Herpetic Eye Disease Study Group. *N Engl J Med* 1998; **339**: 300–6.

Barron BA, Gee L, Hauk WW *et al*. Herpetic Eye Disease Study: a controlled trial of oral acyclovir for herpes simplex stromal keratitis. *Ophthalmology* 1994; **101**: 1871–2.

Chandler JW. Herpes keratitis and the immune system. *Ophthalmic Forum* 1984; **2**: 189.

Cook SD, Hill JH. Herpes simplex virus; molecular biology and the possibility of corneal latency. *Surv Ophthalmol* 1991; **36**: 140–8.

Coster DJ, Wilhelmus KR, Michaud R, Jones BR. A comparison of acyclovir and idoxuridine as treatment for ulcerative herpetic keratitis. *Br J Ophthalmol* 1980; **64**: 763.

Dawson CH, Togni B. Herpes simplex eye infections: clinical manifestations, pathogenesis and management. *Surv Ophthalmol* 1976; **21**: 121–35.

Hendricks RL. An immunologist's view of herpes simplex keratitis. *Cornea* 1997; **16**: 503–6.

Jones BR, Coster DJ, Falcon MG, Cantell K. Topical therapy of ulcerative herpetic keratitis with human interferon. *Lancet* 1976; **2**: 128.

Jones BR, Fison PN, Cobo LM *et al*. Efficacy of acycloguanosine (Wellcome 248U) against herpes-simplex cornea ulcers. *Lancet* 1979; **1**: 243.

Kaufman HE. Clinical cure of herpes simplex keratitis by 5-iodo-2'-deoxyuridine. *Proc Soc Exp Biol Med* 1962; **109**: 251.

Kaufman HE. Epithelial erosion syndrome: metaherpetic keratitis. *Am J Ophthalmol* 1964; **57**: 983.

Kaufman HE, Martola EL, Dohlman CH. Use of 5-iodo-2'-deoxyuridine (IDU) treatment of herpes simplex keratitis. *Arch Ophthalmol* 1962; **68**: 235–9.

Liesegang TJ. Biology and molecular aspects of herpes simplex and varicella-zoster virus infections. *Ophthalmology* 1992; **99**: 781.

Liesegang TJ. Corneal complications from herpes zoster ophthalmicus. *Ophthalmology* 1985; **92**: 316.

Liesegang TJ. Epidemiology of ocular herpes simplex: natural history in Rochester, Minnesota, 1950 through 1982. *Arch Ophthalmol* 1989; **107**: 1160.

Liu T, Tang Q, Hendricks RL. Inflammatory infiltration of the trigeminal ganglion after herpes simplex virus type 1 corneal infection. *J Virol* 1996; **70**: 264–71.

Marsh RJ, Fraunfelder FT, McGill JL. Herpetic corneal epithelial disease. *Arch Ophthalmol* 1976; **94**: 1899.

Marsh RJ. Ophthalmic herpes zoster. *Br J Hosp Med* 1976; **15**: 609.

Moyes AL, Sugar A, Musch DC, Barnes RD. Antiviral therapy after penetrating keratoplasty for herpes simplex keratitis. *Arch Ophthalmol* 1994; **112**: 601.

Nash AA, Cambouropoulos P. The immune response to herpes simplex virus. *Virology* 1993; **4**: 181–6.

Norrild B. Humoral response to herpes simplex virus infections. In: Roizman B, Lopex C, eds. *The Herpesviruses*. New York: Plenum Press, 1985.

Shuster JJ, Kaufman HE, Nesburn AB. Statistical analysis of the rate of recurrence of herpes virus ocular epithelial disease. *Am J Ophthalmol* 1981; **91**: 328.

Streilein JW, Dana MR, Ksander BR. Immunity causing blindness; five different paths to herpes stromal keratitis. *Immunol Today* 1997; **18**: 443–9.

Wellings PC, Awdry PN, Bors FH *et al*. Clinical evaluation of trifluorothymidine in the treatment of herpes simplex cornea ulcers. *Am J Ophthalmol* 1972; **73**: 932.

Wilhelmus KR, Coster DJ, Jones BR. Acyclovir and debridement in the treatment of ulcerative herpetic keratitis. *Am J Ophthalmol* 1981; **91**: 323.

Wilhelmus KR, Gee L, Hauk WW *et al*. Herpetic Eye Disease Study (HEDS): a controlled trial of topical corticosteroids for herpes simplex stromal keratitis. *Ophthalmology* 1994; **101**: 1883.

10 Corneal trauma

Corneal trauma is common. As the most exposed anatomical element of the eye, the cornea is likely to take the brunt of most physical insults directed at the eye.

As part of its protective role, the cornea has evolved into a tough integument capable of withstanding substantial force. It is, however, vulnerable because a normal ultrastructure must be maintained if its function is not to be compromised. The healing response of the cornea, even to trivial insults, may interfere with subsequent optical function.

Furthermore, the protective and optical function of the cornea may be acutely embarrassed by the disruption resulting from trauma. Corneal ulceration may lead to infection, oedema may lead to corneal neovascularisation, and blood staining may be complicated by fibrosis. Prompt and effective management of trauma is needed to prevent secondary damage which may be more threatening to the eye than the initial injury.

The clinical encounter

No two injuries are the same and the extent of damage caused by trauma can be more extensive than may initially appear. Bleeding, anterior chamber angle damage or even a retinal detachment may complicate a corneal abrasion from blunt trauma. As simple as an injury may seem, a complete clinical assessment must be made, although not necessarily in the first instance. The initial assessment must be as complete as possible, particularly the assessment of visual function, but some aspects, such as examination of the retinal periphery, can be delayed until the acute discomfort is over.

At the initial assessment, it is necessary to accurately record the patient's account of how the injury occurred, the visual acuity, and to precisely document the way in which the eye is damaged. Because even trivial corneal injuries can be painful, it is often necessary to instil a drop of local anaesthetic to facilitate clinical assessment.

Irradiation injury to the cornea

Two types of corneal injury due to irradiation are commonly seen: the reaction to ultraviolet light and delayed necrosis as a consequence of therapeutic use of ionising radiation to treat pterygia.

Ultraviolet radiation injury

The cornea is susceptible to damage when exposed to ultraviolet light between 210 and 360 nm because light in this range is preferentially absorbed by nucleic acids and aromatic amino acids. Those likely to suffer ultraviolet injury are welders, skiers, and users of tanning sun lamps (Figure 10.1). Symptoms are severe pain and photophobia 8–12 hours after exposure. It is usually necessary to instil topical local anaesthetic in order to examine the eye with a slit lamp and examination reveals widespread punctate epithelial erosions in the

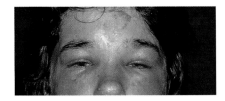

Figure 10.1 Extensive UV burns to periorbital skin and cornea from misguided use of tanning sun lamp

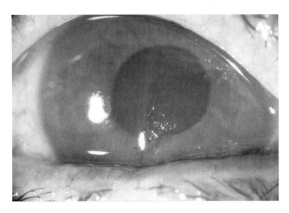

Figure 10.3 Corneal abrasion caused by impact of a tennis ball

exposed area. Spontaneous healing occurs in 24–48 hours without residual visual loss. Treatment is supportive: cycloplegia, tight patching, and oral analgesics.

Ionising radiation injury

In regions where pterygium is common and severe and can threaten visual loss, β irradiation as an adjunct to surgery has been used for many years and has proven very effective. Although there are no obvious acute complications of this use of radiotherapy, there are long term complications. Corneal and scleral necrosis can occur decades after irradiation. When this recalcitrant form of ulceration occurs, it can be complicated by infection which is very threatening to the eye (Figure 10.2).

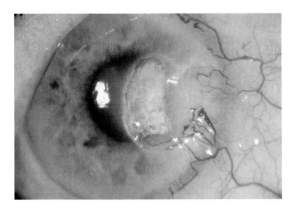

Figure 10.2 Corneoscleral necrosis occurring years after β ray therapy following pterygium excision

Blunt trauma

Blunt trauma may cause a number of injuries to the cornea. Injuries can result from encountering such diverse implements as a boxer's fist or a baby's finger. A common result of blunt trauma to the cornea is an abrasion.

Corneal abrasions

Patients with a corneal abrasion present with a history of trauma and a painful eye (Figure 10.3). The eye is usually so painful that it is necessary to instil local anaesthetic eye drops in order to measure vision and carry out the clinical examination. Corneal abrasions are easily seen with the slit lamp but are more easily seen after rose bengal dye is instilled. Fluorescein is also effective, but rose bengal is preferred because fluorescein stains the stroma and creates a flare in the anterior chamber, making other aspects of the examination more difficult. All the other complications of blunt trauma can occur in patients with a corneal abrasion and must be looked for. These sequelae include hyphaema, angle damage, including angle recession, and retinal damage, including traumatic oedema and even tears. These serious complications will not be found unless they are looked for.

Corneal abrasions occur when the epithelium is stripped off the underlying stroma. Stromal loss is unusual but will become more common as LASIK practice extends (Figure 10.4). The natural history is for healing to occur over 48 hours, even for the largest defects. It takes longer for the repaired epithelium to achieve a stable,

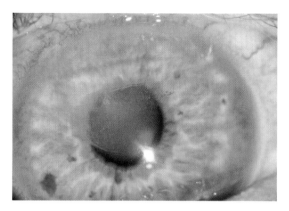

Figure 10.4 Displaced stromal flap in a patient who has had LASIK and suffered minor blunt trauma two years later

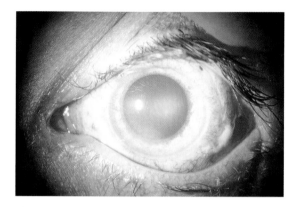

Figure 10.5 Extensive corneal oedema following blunt trauma

fully differentiated histology. Adequate adherence to the underlying basement membrane may not occur for months or even years, resulting in the patient being prone to recurrent erosions.

The aim of treatment is to achieve epithelial healing in the shortest possible time. Nothing can be done to speed healing but it can be impeded, for example, by unnecessary use of topical medication. A low dose of a broad spectrum antibiotic, such as chloramphenicol, is all that is required. A case can be made for avoiding even this, providing close observation of the case is possible.

Supportive measures may also be required because pain and photophobia can be troublesome.

This is best managed by padding the eye until the epithelium has healed. Sometimes oral analgesics are required. Once the epithelium is healed and the eye is comfortable, a more complete examination should be carried out.

Corneal contusion without abrasion

Blunt trauma may cause an abrasion and underlying damage or it may cause corneal injury without necessarily removing the epithelium. This damage may be directly to the cornea or indirect, with the cornea suffering secondary damage as a result of primary damage elsewhere in the eye.

Blunt trauma may cause stromal oedema through direct contusion of the stroma or, as is

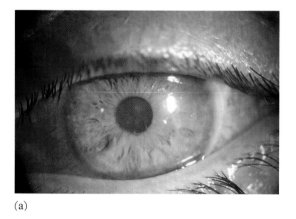

(a)

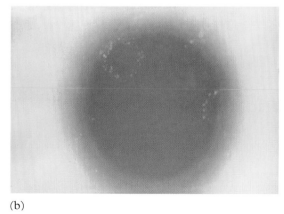

(b)

Figure 10.6 Sand blast injury. (a) Some foreign bodies remain in the superficial cornea, (b) small grey rings are seen at the endothelial level

more often the case, through damage to the corneal endothelium. The endothelium may be injured over a broad area (Figure 10.5) or there may be a multifocal pattern of cell damage (Figure 10.6). The natural history of such an injury is of spontaneous resolution over weeks or months. Observation is all that is required.

Two closed injuries affecting the cornea indirectly are hyphaema and traumatic angle damage (Figure 10.7). Any significant closed trauma can affect the uvea. Haemorrhage from the uvea is common after closed injury to the eye. If hyphaema is complicated by elevated intraocular pressure, blood may leach into the cornea, staining it so that transparency is lost (Figure 10.8). Prevention, by effective management of the primary hyphaema, is the most important strategy. Once blood staining has occurred, a conservative approach is desirable. Blood staining does resolve with time, although this may take months or years.

Blunt trauma to the cornea can be complicated by injury to the anterior chamber angle which, if not recognised, may result in posttraumatic glaucoma threatening vision. Monitoring of intraocular pressure and gonioscopy are mandatory for patients who have had blunt trauma to the eye. If there is a combination of endothelial injury and elevated intraocular pressure, corneal decompensation and corneal oedema frequently occur.

Corneal foreign bodies

The exposed cornea is prone to impaction of foreign bodies. Most are trivial but a few are sight threatening. Dust, sand, or metal blown around in the wind are largely responsible (Figure 10.9).

Patients do not always remember the impaction of the foreign body but present with a painful red eye. Examination reveals the foreign body in the cornea and its nature is usually obvious. When there is inflammation within the corneal stroma, the possibility of infection must be taken seriously. Intraocular penetration and corneal infection are the most serious complications of corneal foreign bodies. Intraocular penetration should be considered if there is suspicion of a high speed projectile. A

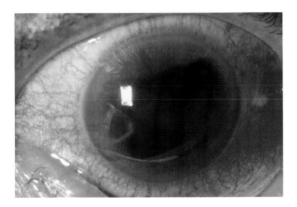

Figure 10.7 Traumatic hyphaema

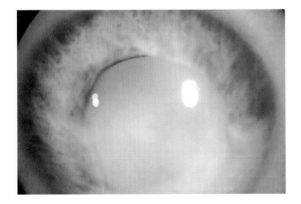

Figure 10.8 Blood staining of the cornea complicating traumatic hyphaema and elevated intraocular pressure

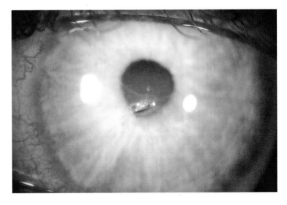

Figure 10.9 Metallic foreign body sustained by factory worker using a grinding wheel

careful history will reveal this possibility. Some types of foreign material are more likely to carry organisms. Vegetable matter is hazardous; bacteria and fungi are often carried on vegetable matter such as wood, leaves, and thorns. Patients who have had these materials in their cornea should be watched carefully.

Corneal foreign bodies should be removed, although occasionally, small biocompatible foreign bodies can be left in the cornea. Exposed material and anything initiating an infection or inducing an inflammatory reaction should be removed.

Removal is carried out at the slit lamp after the installation of topical anaesthetic. This can be done with a hypodermic needle, dental burr or whatever sterile implement is appropriate to remove the foreign body with the least damage to the cornea.

Following removal of the foreign body, patients are given a broad spectrum antibiotic such as chloramphenicol eye drops four times a day and observed regularly until the epithelium has healed, at which time the topical antibiotic can be ceased.

Metal foreign bodies are very commonly picked up in industrial circumstances. There is often leaching of brown rust material into the cornea around embedded metallic foreign bodies, creating a rust ring. This may remain after the foreign body has been removed. The rust ring can be removed at the slit lamp with a 23 gauge hypodermic needle and the case treated subsequently as for other foreign bodies.

Incisional wounds

Incisions made by sharp objects such as knives, glass, and metals are potentially threatening to vision (Figure 10.10). If the cornea is breached, irreparable damage may be done to underlying structures and, at the very least, a portal of entry is created for micro-organisms. Patients who have sustained incisional trauma to the eye demand very careful evaluation. The full extent of the injury must be appreciated, preferably before reparative surgery is undertaken.

Full thickness corneal wounds need exploration and repair, at which time any

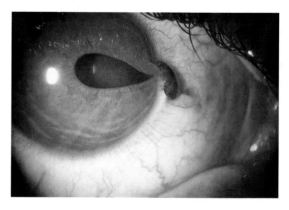

Figure 10.10   Corneoscleral laceration sustained in a stabbing

associated damage, such as iris incarceration or lens damage, should be dealt with. Surgery of traumatic corneal wounds can be demanding because accurate anatomical repair is necessary if visual loss is to be minimised. Microsurgical repair under general anaesthesia is usually required. Even with apparently precise repair, subsequent visual loss can occur.

Small, partial thickness wounds that are not associated with corneal distortion can be left to heal without surgical intervention, providing they are not gaping. Even small partial thickness corneal wounds can result in astigmatism. It was early observations on the refractive effects of corneal trauma that led to the suggestion of incisional surgery for developmental astigmatism.

Penetrating injuries of the globe are a medical emergency. Patients with such injuries require prompt assessment and alleviation of any pain (but not with a drug such as morphine, which may induce vomiting), alleviation of any nausea with an antiemetic, protection of the eye with a shield, antitetanus and antimicrobial prophylaxis. Restorative surgery can wait for up to 12 hours for optimal conditions and is best done early rather than late, providing conditions are optimal.

Tetanus prophylaxis

Almost invariably corneal wounds fall into the category of clean, minor wounds. Such patients should be given active immunisation only if their immunisation history is unknown, if they have had less than three doses of tetanus toxoid through their life, or if their last booster was more than 10 years previously. There is never an indication for passive immunisation with tetanus immune globulin unless the corneal wound is part of more extensive injuries considered to be a high risk for tetanus.

Antimicrobial prophylaxis

All patients with penetrating ocular trauma should receive systemic antimicrobial prophylaxis. They should have an IV line inserted at presentation and intravenous therapy given for at least 72 hours. An aminoglycoside and a second generation cephalosporin provide appropriate coverage.

Post-traumatic endothelial decompensation

The corneal endothelium has limited capacity for repair. When endothelial cells are injured and lost, surrounding cells enlarge and slide to cover the defect. When this occurs, the corneal oedema developing immediately after the injury resolves. If the extent of damage is too great to repair in this way, the corneal oedema persists. Even when resolution does occur, the process of endothelial repair may take many months and the oedema persist accordingly.

With the passage of time, the loss of endothelial cells continues as it does in normal individuals, although the rate of loss is greater in patients who have suffered endothelial damage. Once the endothelial cell count has reduced to less than 1000 cells/mm^2, corneal oedema can occur (see Figure 1.39). This may not happen until some years after the original injury. At first, the oedema is confined to the stroma but as the condition progresses, the epithelium becomes involved. This results in the formation of blisters or bullae. These lesions are painful, especially when the blisters rupture to expose nerve endings. Penetrating corneal transplantation is the only curative procedure for corneal oedema

due to endothelial cell damage. Surgery is the most common cause of direct endothelial injury, cell loss and corneal oedema.

Chemical burns

Alkali, acids, and various oxidising agents can be very threatening to the cornea. Although the clinical effects from exposure of the cornea to various strong chemicals may be different, the general principles of management are similar in all cases.

Alkali burns

Alkali injuries are unfortunately common, serious, and often blinding. Chemicals which can produce an alkali injury include sodium hydroxide, potassium hydroxide, calcium hydroxide, magnesium hydroxide, and ammonium hydroxide.

Alkali injuries are particularly severe because they cause saponification of lipids in cell membranes, which kills cells very effectively and removes any barrier to deeper penetration. Hydroxide ions also irreparably denature proteins such as collagen and glycosaminoglycans. This accounts for the damaging effect of alkalis on blood vessels. Corneal injury by alkali can affect the epithelium, stroma, endothelium, and pericorneal vasculature (Figure 10.11).

The major clinical signs of injury by alkali are epithelial loss, stromal opacification, and limbal ischaemia (Figure 10.12). Adjacent structures such as the lids and conjunctiva may also be affected, as may internal structures of the eye, in particular the iris, the lens, which may become cataractous, and the drainage angle, the result being elevated intraocular pressure. The extent of initial damage judged on epithelial damage, stromal opacification, and limbal ischaemia correlates well with the ultimate prognosis. Corneal alkali burns are classified on the basis of the extent of initial damage and this correlates well with subsequent outcome (Table 10.1). A common sequela of even mild to moderate alkali

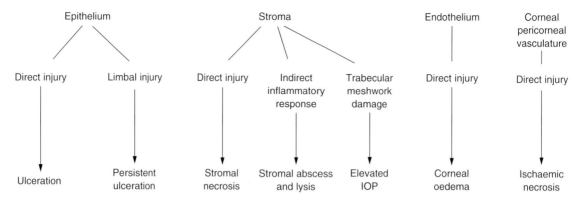

Figure 10.11   Effects of alkali on the cornea

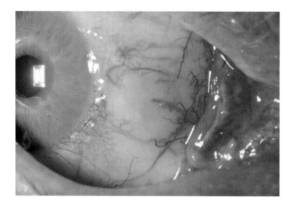

Figure 10.12   Alkali burn of mild to moderate severity. There is epithelial loss, mild stromal opacity, and limbal ischaemia

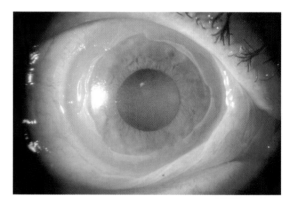

Figure 10.13   Failed epithelial healing after an alkali burn

Table 10.1   Simplified classification of alkali injuries to the eye

	Mild	Moderate	Severe
Epithelial damage	←	All cases	→
Stromal haze	Minimal, iris details can be seen	Moderate, iris details blurred	Pupil barely visible or not seen
Perilimbal ischaemia	None	$<\frac{1}{2}$	$>\frac{1}{2}$

burns is failure of the corneal epithelium to heal (Figure 10.13).

Acid burns

Acid burns can be as serious for the eye as alkali burns and demand similar vigilance and comprehensive care. Acids tend to coagulate and precipitate corneal proteins. The extent of damage caused is related to the pH and the affinity of the anion for the corneal proteins. Acids tend to fix tissues and this may limit the extent of damage so that it is not as great as it might be with alkali burns of similar severity. However, with severe acid burns, damage may be every bit as severe as that seen with severe alkali burns.

Acid burns should be carefully assessed and graded on the same basis as alkali burns.

Burns from oxidising agents

Various organic oxidising agents, such as methyl ethylmethyl ketone peroxide used in fibreglass manufacture and Paraquat in agriculture, can produce blinding disruption of

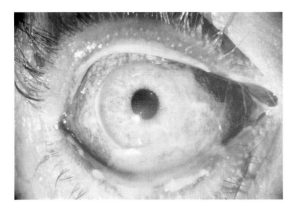

Figure 10.14 Paraquat injury in an agricultural worker

the cornea. With these cases, tissue damage with inflammation and fibrosis can proceed for months and years after the initial injury, as if the agent has become bound to ocular tissues (Figure 10.14).

The initial treatment of these cases is similar to that for alkali burns, but anti-inflammatory therapy may be necessary for months or years.

Treatment of chemical injuries to the cornea

The emergency treatment of alkali injuries involves immediate lavage of the eye at the time and place of injury. Most of the damage is done in seconds and minutes so that immediate lavage can alleviate damage. In the accident and emergency department, further lavage should be carried out with sterile balanced salt solution if the injury has occurred within two hours of presentation.

Any particulate matter should be removed from the surface of the eye and the conjunctival sac. This can be done with a cotton tipped applicator.

In addition, any fibrinous debris should be removed with sterile microsurgical forceps. This is not usually present at the time of the injury but accumulates over the next few days and perhaps weeks.

Pupil dilation is desirable to prevent troublesome posterior synechiae. One drop of atropine 1% per day is appropriate for this purpose.

The intraocular pressure may rise to unacceptable levels and this is best managed with systemic carbonic anhydrase inhibitors. Topical agents such as β blockers are also effective but it is desirable to avoid topical medication wherever possible. Poor epithelial healing and persistent epithelial defects are common and disastrous sequelae of chemical burns, particularly alkali burns. Nothing can be done to facilitate epithelial healing, but it is very easy to retard epithelial healing with topical medication.

For this reason topical medication is best avoided in patients with chemical burns unless there is a definite indication and confirmed benefit has been demonstrated in appropriate studies. For this reason, topical antibiotics may be best avoided if the patient is sensible and compliant and close observation and supervision by an ophthalmologist are possible.

After the acute phase, more chronic problems persist or develop. Persistant ulceration, symblepharon formation, inflammation and vascularisation of the cornea, cicatricial entropion, trichiasis, and glaucoma may be troublesome. Each must be treated on its merits. It is important when treating these conditions to avoid excessive topical medication and to avoid unnecessary trauma from "glass rodding" the fornices and other such manoeuvres, the benefits of which have not been proven. The use of some drugs, which have been shown to be beneficial in animal experiments, remain experimental in clinical practice. Acetyl cysteine and L-cysteine, two agents with anticollagenase activity, and scorbic acid are currently being assessed in clinical trials. So too is the use of amniotic membrane in the acute post-injury phase.

Rehabilitation after chemical injuries is challenging. Conventional corneal transplantation has a very high failure rate when done to restore vision to those with corneal scarring from chemical burns. Limbal damage, which limits epithelial healing and differentiation, is largely responsible for the poor outcome. Limbal transplantation offers some prospect of overcoming this problem.

Corneal injury from surgery

Intraocular surgery is the most common cause of serious corneal injury. Many surgical procedures are carried out within, or in close proximity to, the cornea and the structure is vulnerable to injury and limited in its capacity to repair. Some injuries have serious implications, others are more transient. Many of the injuries suffered by the cornea during surgery are avoidable.

Epithelial loss

Loss of corneal epithelium can occur during surgery or in the early postoperative period. At the time of surgery, inadvertent injury may occur or it may be necessary to remove the epithelium in order to obtain a better view of the intraocular structures. Topical medication given prior to or during surgery can result in impaired epithelial transparency and the only way to deal with this effectively is to remove the epithelium. This can be done gently with a soft instrument such as a cellulose sponge.

In the postoperative period, corneal ulceration may occur because the lids have not been adequately closed at the end of the procedure or, in some cases, cannot be closed, so that the cornea is left exposed and prone to epithelial desiccation. The preferred management is avoidance and this can be done with due care. Occasionally, a foreign body left under the tarsis can cause ulceration or there may be long suture ends between the lid and the corneal epithelium.

Toxic epitheliopathy

Topical medications used before and during surgery, such as dilating drops, can result in epithelial toxicity. This may take the form of punctate epithelial erosions or, if the use of medication is prolonged, may be seen as punctate keratopathy but in the acute phase there is usually a diffuse loss of corneal epithelial transparency. Again, the best treatment is preventive, in particular, not to overmedicate and to avoid commonly used agents known to be toxic to the corneal epithelium, such as phenylephrine.

Postsurgical superior limbic keratitis and filamentary keratitis

In the postoperative period, the relationship between the epithelium and the tear film can be disturbed. The combination of excess mucus and abnormal epithelium can result in the formation of filaments, aggregations of mucus on disturbed epithelium which can pull the epithelium from its underlying support structures, causing considerable pain. The cause of this is multifactorial. The epithelium is often abnormal after surgery so that it is not fully differentiated, creating mucus receptors. In addition, tear secretion may be reduced and, if there is inflammation, the mucus secretion may be increased. Filaments may occur all over the cornea but sometimes they are confined to the superior cornea in the vicinity of the limbus. There are at least three factors operating to produce superior limbic keratoconjunctivitis: an abnormal epithelium which contains mucus receptors, abnormal tear movement, and an abnormal "shear relationship" between the upper lid and the globe. Postoperative superior limbic keratitis is similar to that which occurs spontaneously.

Microbial keratitis

Microbial keratitis may complicate ocular surgery. Following surgery, the normal defence mechanisms of the cornea are compromised in a number of ways. The incision provides a portal of entry for organisms, suture material provides a foreign body nidus which encourages infection, antibiotics may encourage the overgrowth of pathogenic strains and topical corticosteroids, given to decrease postoperative inflammation, may decrease normal host resistance to infection. Most microbial keratitis complicating surgery occurs in relationship to sutures. It should be managed along the lines set out in the relevant section on corneal ulceration.

Dellen formation

A dellen is a focal area of stromal dehydration. These lesions tend to occur beside elevated areas of cornea where the normal irrigation system of the mobile lid and tear film is disturbed by a focal high spot. A dellen is invariably temporary unless corneal ulceration occurs. Under these circumstances, there can be local necrosis and the cornea is exposed to an increased risk of infection.

Descemet's membrane detachment

Descemet's membrane may be detached at the time of surgery. This is a more common problem since the use of small incisions has become the method of choice for common procedures such as cataract surgery. Descemet's membrane can be pushed away from the surrounding stroma at the time of the introduction of instruments through tight incisions. Small detachments are of no consequence but larger detachments can be associated with epithelial oedema. The treatment of these lesions is to reattach them with either a viscoelastic material or air, with the patient subsequently positioned in the immediate postoperative period to ensure that the air bubble pushes the Descemet's membrane back into position.

Endothelial cell loss

Endothelial cell loss occurs after all anterior segment surgery and can be sufficient to cause corneal oedema. After corneal endothelial trauma with cell loss, repair is by endothelial cell slide and enlargement. This is reflected in the endothelial cell count. If the endothelial cell count falls below 1000 cells per square millimetre, then corneal oedema is likely to occur.

In general, the more traumatic the operation, the more extensive the endothelial cell loss. A feature of the progress of ocular microsurgery is decreasing endothelial trauma. With modern cataract surgery, endothelial cell loss in uncomplicated cases is below 5%. After uncomplicated corneal transplantation surgery with a successful visual outcome, endothelial cell counts may be 30–50%.

The most effective management of endothelial cell loss at the time of surgery is preventive. Careful microsurgery with the use of protective viscoelastic material is mandatory if the complication of bullous keratopathy is to be minimised and, preferably, avoided.

Bullous keratopathy often does not occur for many years after the original surgery. This is because the normal rate of cell loss with age is accelerated after surgery.

The only treatment for endothelial cell loss causing corneal oedema is corneal transplantation with a penetrating graft.

Cell loss suffered by patients having anterior segment surgery occurs at the time of surgery. For patients with intraocular lenses, cell loss may be aggravated in subsequent years by the malpositioning of the lens in the anterior chamber or clipped to the iris. Continuing cell loss is minimal, with modern intraocular lenses being placed within the capsular bag with an intact capsulorhexis.

Corneal wound derangement

Wound dehiscence

The most common corneal wound complication is dehiscence. Corneal wound healing is slow because of the relatively acellular nature of the cornea; it takes many months for corneal wounds to regain anything like normal corneal strength. Care must be taken not to remove corneal sutures prematurely. In adults, corneal transplant sutures should remain in place for a year. In children, corneal wounds heal much more rapidly and suture removal can be carried out after corneal grafts within months.

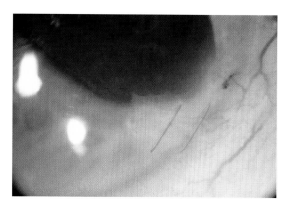

Figure 10.15 Epithelial downgrowth after repair of penetrating limbal injury

Epithelial downgrowth

Epithelium may grow through the wound and onto the back of the cornea (Figure 10.15). Epithelial downgrowths are very unusual today because of the precise nature of corneal microsurgery. This has not always been the case and, in some unusual circumstances, epithelial downgrowths are encountered even today. Effective treatment is difficult. The downgrowth should be excised and there are advocates for cryotherapy of the surrounding area, although this is a very non-specific approach which induces considerable collateral damage.

Astigmatism

Astigmatism is so common as to be almost universal after corneal wounds, even small ones. Astigmatism after corneal wounds occurs for two broad reasons. First, corneal tissue is more compressible than it is stretchable. Because it is so inelastic, tight sutures distort the corneal shape by compressing it within tight loops and creating distortion elsewhere in the cornea. Second, the fibrosis of wound healing is a highly variable entity. Wound dehiscence short of rupture, and due to weak wound healing, is relatively common. In other cases, where there is excessive fibrosis, the effect of this is similar to what has been described with tight suture loops, so that distortion remote from the wound itself occurs, creating astigmatism.

The treatment of astigmatism depends on its origin. Irregular astigmatism is best dealt with by the use of a contact lens. This is also a very good test of the contribution of irregular astigmatism to visual loss. A hard contact lens negates the irregular astigmatism and, if it is the only factor contributing to visual loss, the increase in acuity is striking. With high levels of regular astigmatism, incisional techniques are appropriate.

Further reading

Bourne WM, Kaufman HE. Cataract extraction and the corneal endothelium. *Am J Ophthalmol* 1976; **82**: 44.

Broderick JD. Corneal blood staining after hyphaema. *Br J Ophthalmol* 1972; **56**: 589.

Cibis GW, Weingeist TA, Krachmer JH. Traumatic corneal endothelial rings. *Arch Ophthalmol* 1978; **96**: 485.

Eisner G. *Eye Surgery*. New York: Springer Verlag, 1990.

Flynn CA, D'Amico F, Smith G. Should we patch corneal abrasions? A meta-analysis. *J Fam Pract* 1998; **47**: 264–70.

Forstot SL, Gasset AR. Transient traumatic posterior annular keratopathy of Payrau. *Arch Ophthalmol* 1974; **92**: 527.

Foulks GN, Friend J, Thoft RA. Effects of ultraviolet radiation on corneal epithelial metabolism. *Invest Ophthalmol Vis Sci* 1978; **17**: 694.

Grant WM, Schuman JS. *Toxicology of the eye*, 4th edn. Springfield: Charles C Thomas, 1993.

Hirst LW, Smiddy WE, DeJuan E. Tissue adhesive therapy for corneal perforations. *Aust J Ophthalmol* 1983; **11**: 113–18.

Pfister RR. The effects of chemical injury on the ocular surface. *Ophthalmology* 1983; **90**: 601.

Ringvold A, Davanger M, Olsen EG. Changes of the corneal epithelium after ultraviolet radiation. *Acta Ophthalmol (Copenh)* 1982; **60**: 41.

Van Rij G, Waring GO. Changes in corneal curvature induced by sutures and incisions. *Am J Ophthalmol* 1984; **98**: 773.

Vastine DW, Weinberg RS, Sugar J *et al*. Stripping of Descemet's membrane associated with intraocular lens implantation. *Arch Ophthalmol* 1983; **101**: 1042.

Waltman SR, Cozean CH, Jr. The effect of phacoemulsification on the corneal endothelium. *Ophthalmic Surg* 1979; **10**: 31.

Wessels IF, McNeill JI. Applicator for cyanoacrylate tissue adhesive. *Ophthalmic Surg* 1989; **80**: 211–14.

11 Corneal dystrophies

The corneal dystrophies are a group of conditions which affect the cornea and share some striking clinical features. In particular, they are inherited bilateral conditions and are confined to the cornea. Not all conditions considered to be corneal dystrophies conform precisely to this pattern, but most do. All corneal dystrophies are rare and most are very rare; Fuchs' dystrophy is the only dystrophy encountered at all commonly in clinical practice. All dystrophies have striking clinical appearances but these may differ from one to another, even within what is considered to be the same condition, and sometimes between family members afflicted with a particular dystrophy. Usually both eyes are affected in a symmetrical manner but even this is not invariable; some patients have considerably more morphological change in one eye than the other. This is often the case with Fuchs' dystrophy and sometimes the case with lattice dystrophy.

In recent years, a better understanding of the underlying biochemical basis for dystrophies has developed and for some the genetic defect has been identified. An understanding of the genetic basis of the disorders may provide some surprising insights. For example, lattice dystrophy and granular dystrophy, two conditions with quite different clinical appearances, have recently been shown to have the identical genetic mutation.

A more complete understanding of the genetic basis of corneal dystrophies may also lead to an improved classification of the disorders but for the time being they are classified on an anatomical and morphological basis. The accepted classification divides the dystrophies into epithelial, stromal, and endothelial groups, with each group further subdivided on the basis of the morphological changes apparent at a clinical level.

Corneal dystrophies produce symptoms in a number of ways. Corneal transparency may be affected adversely by the accumulation of metabolic products in the normally clear corneal stroma, as occurs with macular dystrophy. Some patients develop recurrent erosions which eventually lead to corneal scarring and loss of transparency, as is the case with anterior membrane dystrophies, Reis–Bückler's, lattice dystrophy, and, sometimes, with granular dystrophy. Corneal transparency may also be reduced by oedema, as occurs with Fuchs' dystrophy, congenital endothelial dystrophy and, occasionally, with posterior polymorphous dystrophy.

The clinical diagnosis is based on the slit lamp appearances. Usually these are quite characteristic.

The histological appearances are also characteristic, but as a minority of patients come to corneal transplantation, histological examination is usually useful only in retrospect after a patient has required corneal transplantation. With identification of the genetic basis of an increasing number of dystrophies, it is usually wise to look specifically for the relevant mutation, particularly if the dystrophy is clinically significant, unusual in clinical features or if genetic counselling is required.

The essential features of dystrophies likely to be encountered in routine practice are set out in Table 11.1. Undoubtedly there are dystrophies which are not yet classified. This is particularly obvious when working in genetically distinct communities, such as in some isolated geographic regions and where medical disorders are less well documented. In such a situation, there is an opportunity to document undescribed conditions. Some of the more commonly encountered dystrophies found in Western communities deserve further description.

Superficial dystrophies

Anterior membrane dystrophy

A number of conditions affecting the superficial cornea can be considered to be dystrophic and are probably related. These include inherited recurrent erosion dystrophy, map dot dystrophy and anterior membrane dystrophy. Perhaps these terms describe the same process. Common to these dystrophies is a propensity to recurrent erosion and the

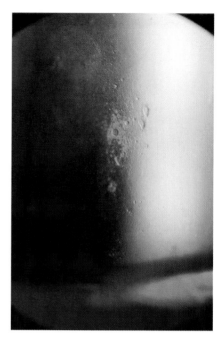

Figure 11.1 Microcysts in the corneal epithelium. Similar lesions may result from dystrophic changes, epithelial healing after ulceration, and contact lens wear

occurrence of cysts (Figure 11.1) and lines (Figure 11.2), either fine lines or broader lines, in the epithelial and subepithelial regions.

Table 11.1   Essential features of dystrophies likely to be encountered in routine clinical practice

Dystrophy	Inheritance	Gene locus	Biochemical abnormality
Superficial			
Reis–Bückler's	Autosomal dominant	5q31	Fibrovascular replacement of Bowman's layer
Meesmann's	Autosomal dominant	12q and 17q	Cytokeratin abnormality
Anterior membrane/map dot/recurrent erosion	Autosomal dominant	Unknown	Undefined abnormalities of epithelial adherence
Stromal			
Schnyder's central crystalline	Autosomal dominant	1p34.1 1-p36	Cholesterol
Granular	Autosomal dominant	5q22-q32	Electron dense deposits of unknown composition
Lattice:			
type I	Autosomal dominant	5q22-q32	Amyloid
type II	Autosomal dominant	9q34	Amyloid
type III	Autosomal recessive	Unknown	Amyloid
type IIIA	Autosomal dominant	Unknown	Amyloid
Macular	Autosomal recessive	16q21	Glycosaminoglycans
Posterior			
Congenital endothelial	Autosomal recessive	Unknown	Oedema
Fuchs'	Autosomal dominant	Unknown	Oedema and collagenous thickening behind Descemet's membrane
Posterior polymorphous	Autosomal dominant	20q12-q13.1	Abnormal Descemet's membrane

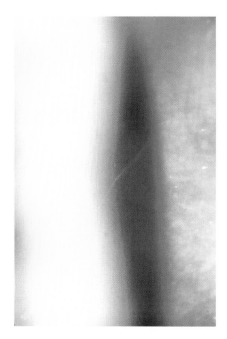

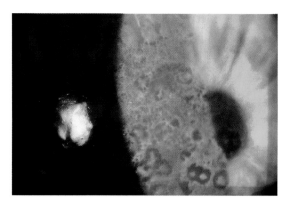

Figure 11.3 Reis–Bückler's dystrophy. There is a diffuse opacity at the level of Bowman's membrane which is honeycombed and incomplete

Figure 11.2 Fine fibrillary line in a patient with anterior membrane dystrophy

The broad lines seen in these patients probably represent the edge of previous erosions where there has been some fibrosis, much like a beach around a lake. The fine lines, however, and the cysts are more likely to be indicative of poorly adherent epithelium. The nature of the essential pathology is unknown.

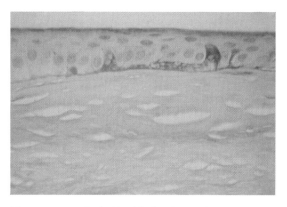

Figure 11.4 Reis–Bückler's dystrophy. Bowman's membrane is replaced by fibrovascular material with a fibrillary nature

Reis–Bückler's dystrophy

Reis–Bückler's dystrophy is a relatively common condition in which the pathology is related to Bowman's membrane. There is diffuse opacity observable at the slit lamp which is often honeycombed and incomplete (Figure 11.3). The normal Bowman's membrane is replaced by fibrovascular material with a fibrillary nature (Figure 11.4). The overlying epithelium is inadequately adherent and prone to recurrent erosion; once this occurs, scarring is common and this is often a significant contributing factor to decreasing vision. Surgery may be required. In the past, lamellar or even penetrating keratoplasties have been preferred for this

condition. Although reasonably successful, however, recurrence in the graft is well known. More recently, therapeutic keratectomy using an excimer laser has been advocated but the value of this approach is yet to be verified.

Stromal dystrophies

The three most commonly encountered stromal dystrophies are granular (Figure 11.5), lattice (Figure 11.6), and macular (Figure 11.7) dystrophies. Granular and lattice dystrophy are dominantly inherited while macular dystrophy is recessively inherited. Macular dystrophy is, therefore, more common in communities with

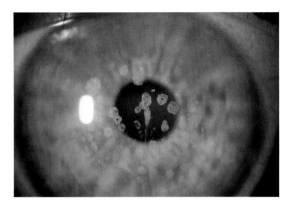

Figure 11.5 Granular dystrophy. Small discrete opacities are seen in the stroma and the intervening stroma has normal transparency

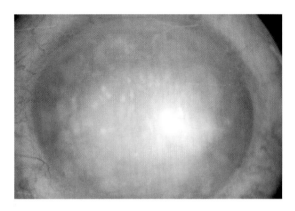

Figure 11.7 Macular dystrophy. Focal opacities are seen in the stroma and the intervening stroma is opaque

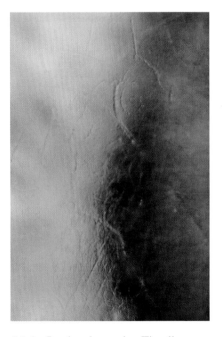

Figure 11.6 Lattice dystrophy. Fine linear opacities are seen in the stroma. The intervening stroma has normal transparency

higher levels of consanguinity. The essential features of these disorders are set out in Table 11.2. In recent years, it has been appreciated that lattice dystrophy occurs in a number of forms; it has been classified as occurring in type I, II, III, and IIIA forms. All these are dominantly inherited, apart from type III which is recessively inherited. Type I or classic lattice

dystrophy is much more common than the other three subtypes.

Another rare stromal dystrophy is Avellino dystrophy which has typical superficial granular lesions and fusiform amyloid deposits in the deeper stromal layers. Recently it has been shown that granular, lattice, and Avellino dystrophy have the same genetic mutation.

Endothelial dystrophies

Fuchs' dystrophy

Fuchs' dystrophy is a relatively common disorder, at least when compared to other corneal dystrophies. The essential pathology is a deficiency in the corneal endothelium; the endothelial cell count decreases below normal values and eventually stromal and epithelial oedema ensue. Abnormalities of Descemet's membrane arise in association with reduplications and foci of thickening; slit lamp examination reveals the same features seen histologically. Corneal oedema, local thickenings of Descemet's membrane, described as guttatae, and endothelial abnormalities are readily seen in most cases (Figure 11.8). Nuclear cataracts also occur in patients with Fuchs' dystrophy but are not consistently present; sometimes they are absent, sometimes they are advanced at the time of presentation. Patients troubled by Fuchs'

Table 11.2 Features of the three commonly encountered stromal dystrophies

Clinical features	Granular dystrophy	Macular dystrophy	Lattice dystrophy
Heredity	Autosomal dominant	Autosomal recessive	Autosomal dominant
Age of onset			
Signs	1st decade	1st decade	1st decade
Symptoms	3rd decade or later, if at all	2nd decade	2nd–3rd decade
Visual disability	4th–5th decade, if at all	2nd or 3rd decade	2nd–3rd decade
Spontaneous erosions	Uncommon	Common	Very common
Opacities	Discrete with clear stroma between Clear limbal zone	Discrete but with opaque stroma between Limbal zone involved	Linear, but with minor degree of opacity between lines Limbal zone clear
Stromal accumulations	Phospholipids and fibrillar material	Glycosaminoglycans	Amyloid
Treatment (if indicated)	Seldom required (does recur in grafts)	Corneal transplantation (does recur in grafts)	Corneal transplantation (recurs more commonly than with granular or macular)

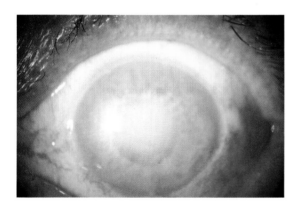

Figure 11.8 Fuchs' dystrophy. Corneal oedema occurs invariably in time. Irregular thickenings of Bowman's membrane are apparent before the appearance of oedema

dystrophy complain of poor vision. If this is due to endothelial failure and oedema, vision is particularly poor in the morning but tends to clear over hours. Marginal endothelial function is further compromised by corneal hypoxia which occurs under closed-eye conditions of sleep. The time it takes for vision to clear in the morning is a measure of corneal compromise and a convenient way to follow the progress of the condition.

Pain occurs in advanced cases due to bullae forming in oedematous epithelium. Epithelial oedema comes later, after the stroma is overhydrated and unable to hold any more water.

A coincidental cataract, which is a common accompaniment of the corneal changes, can also adversely affect vision. It is important to determine the relative contributions of the cornea and the lenticular components of the disease to visual loss, as this must be taken into account if surgical intervention is required. The essential question here is whether the cataract needs to be removed.

Treatment is surgical. Various temporising measures to reduce the impact of corneal oedema, such as promoting evaporation with a hair dryer and the use of hypertonic eye drops, can be tried. However, the therapeutic imperative is for a new corneal endothelium. At present this can only be achieved with a penetrating corneal graft. Because of the rate of complications and the steady increase of complications occurring over time, surgery should be reserved for patients with significant disability.

The failure rate of corneal grafts done for Fuchs' dystrophy is higher than it is for other dystrophies, but not as high as it is for patients having corneal transplants for inflammatory disorders such as herpetic keratitis. Added to the usual risk of allograft rejection, which is a little higher in Fuchs' than other dystrophies, there is another form of graft failure which is not common in grafts done for other conditions. Insidious endothelial failure can occur with time and be associated with the re-establishment of oedema in the cornea.

It is now clear that late endothelial failure also occurs. Corneal endothelium on the graft is not replaced with host endothelium. This is quite different to what happens with epithelium and stromal keratocytes; the former is replaced with host epithelial cells in a matter of weeks or months and the stromal cells are replaced within months or years. After all full thickness grafts the rate of endothelial cell loss is greater than occurs in the normal cornea but after corneal transplantation for Fuchs' dystrophy the rate of cell loss is greater again than the loss occurring in grafts done for other dystrophic conditions. This increased rate of endothelial cell loss is not the only post-transplant observation in those with Fuchs' dystrophy, but is difficult to explain. Patients with Fuchs' dystrophy also have more wound healing problems; dehiscence after suture removal is more common with Fuchs' patients than with any other group. This is puzzling in a condition considered to affect the corneal endothelium, without any obvious abnormality elsewhere in the cornea.

Corneal transplantation is reserved for patients sufficiently disabled to warrant exposure to the risk of surgery. Since the disorder primarily affects the endothelium only a penetrating corneal graft will do. A common issue is what to do about any cataract present at the time of surgery. Should the patient have a cataract removal and an intraocular lens inserted at the time of graft or should there be two operations? If the patient has poor vision at the time of transplantation and a well developed cataract, a combined approach is justified. If,

however, there is mild to moderate cataract, this is best left to be dealt with when it becomes a problem. This may be never or it may be soon after transplantation surgery. The advantage of a two-stage procedure is that the refractive result can be more carefully controlled. Anisometropia and astigmatism are common after corneal transplantation and can be corrected with careful selection of the intraocular lens power. Whether the patient has a staged procedure or a combined procedure does not influence graft survival. Apart from the issues related to the management of cataract, patients having corneal grafts for Fuchs' dystrophy are managed in the same way as anyone else having a penetrating corneal graft.

Treatment of other dystrophies

Corneal transplantation remains the only means of achieving normal corneal function for those adversely affected by corneal dystrophies. This procedure is more effective for some dystrophies than for others. For example, epithelial dystrophies recur quickly in a graft, so quickly that transplantation is not advocated, whilst stromal dystrophies also recur in the graft, but more slowly. Penetrating corneal transplantation is at its most effective in treating these disorders. One problem patients encounter, however, is the recurrence of the dystrophic process in the graft; this tends to occur more quickly with some dystrophies than with others. Lattice dystrophy, in particular, recurs quickly, but so too can macular and granular dystrophy. The allograft rejection rate that is seen with patients having transplants for acquired inflammatory disorders does not occur in patients having grafts for dystrophies, nor is there the same degree of postoperative astigmatism as occurs in patients with ectatic disorders, such as keratoconus. Patients having corneal transplantation for stromal or endothelial dystrophies require a standard penetrating graft and seldom need any associated procedures.

In recent times, excimer laser phototherapeutic keratoplasty (PTK) has been advocated for the treatment of superficial dystrophies, including the epithelial dystrophies prone to recurrent erosions, such as Reis–Bückler's dystrophy. Although strongly advocated by some, the results have been disappointing and the procedure must be considered to be under development.

The only other treatment that needs to be considered is that for recurrent erosions in those with superficial dystrophies. As with recurrent erosions in other situations, the aim of treatment is to establish re-epithelialisation as soon as possible, thereby reducing the risk of infection and the chance of scarring. Nothing can be done to facilitate healing but much can be done to impede it. In particular, the use of topical medications without strong indication may both hinder re-epithelialisation and encourage scarring. The use of eye pads is a time honoured method of encouraging re-epithelialisation but there is no evidence that they actually do so. They do, however, reduce the pain, which can be severe in patients with an acute erosion.

In patients with recurrent erosions, it is important to appreciate the presence of any underlying dystrophy as early as possible. If the true nature of the condition is not understood, it is possible that patients will be misdiagnosed and treated inappropriately. For example, patients with subtle superficial dystrophies are sometimes thought to be suffering from recurrent dendritic keratitis and are treated with antivirals, which slow healing and increase scarring. Accurate diagnosis is important, even if it does not lead to a specific treatment and especially if it means the avoidance of unhelpful therapeutic intervention.

Iridocorneal endothelial syndrome

Iridocorneal endothelial (ICE) syndrome is not a dystrophy, but this rare condition has a similar clinical appearance to corneal dystrophies and hence is included here.

This curious condition was first described in various reports in the early 1900s as essential (or progressive) iris atrophy, often associated with

elevated intraocular pressure (IOP) (Figure 11.9). Chandler reported patients with abnormal corneal endothelium and corneal oedema, which occurred with minimal elevations of IOP (Chandler's syndrome) (Figure 11.10) and Cogan and Reece reported cases of pigmented iris nodules, corneal oedema, and elevated IOP (Cogan–Reece syndrome) (Figure 11.11).

Because iris and corneal endothelial abnormalities are common to these various clinical expressions, the conditions are grouped as iridocorneal endothelial syndrome, or ICE syndrome, which coincidentally is also an acronym for the commonly used terms of iris

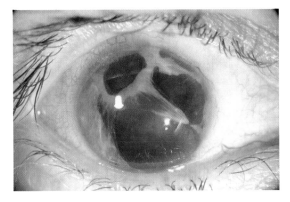

Figure 11.9 Essential iris atrophy. Areas of focal iris atrophy are apparent. In more advanced cases these defects may become full thickness, the pupil distorted, and peripheral anterior synechiae develop

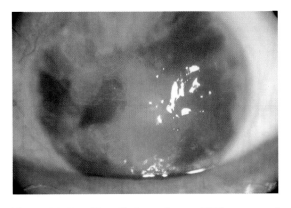

Figure 11.10 Chandler's syndrome. Diffuse corneal oedema is well advanced in this case. There were also some areas of iris atrophy and peripheral anterior synechiae

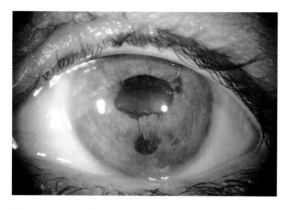

Figure 11.11 Cogan–Reece syndrome. There is mild corneal oedema, dark elevated nodes on the iris surface, and peripheral anterior synechiae

naevus syndrome, Chandler's syndrome and essential iris atrophy.

Clinical features

Patients present with decreased vision due to corneal oedema or may notice asymmetry of the pupils due to iris atrophy. The most common reason for presentation is corneal oedema, so that the condition is often mistaken for an endothelial corneal dystrophy. A summary of conditions which can be confused with ICE syndrome is shown in Table 11.3.

In a fully expressed case, slit lamp examination reveals iris atrophy and naevi or abnormal corneal endothelium, peripheral anterior synechiae, and elevated IOP. The clinical features of ICE and other conditions which have

similar findings are set out in Table 11.4. Since the condition progresses slowly over years, the patient may present early with minimal changes.

Pathology

The corneal stroma is usually oedematous and often inflamed; however, it is the endothelium which is of particular interest. Usually, the endothelial cells are attenuated and pleomorphic. In some cases, the endothelium has been described as epithelialisation of the endothelium with surface microvilli, cell membrane blebs, and abnormal intracellular borders. Transmission electron microscopy reveals a banded or fibrillary layer between the endothelium and Descemet's membrane. The

Table 11.4   Clinical features of ICE syndrome which occur in other conditions

Clinical feature	Possible cause
Corneal oedema	Fuchs' endothelial dystrophy Post-traumatic endothelial failure Posterior polymorphous dystrophy
Iris defects	Ischaemic atrophy Axenfeld–Reiger's syndrome Aniridia Iridoschisis
Iris nodules	Neoplasia Neurofibromatosis

Angle abnormalities	Peripheral anterior synechiae:
	    trauma
	    uveitis
	Neovascular glaucoma
	Trauma

Table 11.3   Conditions which can be confused with iridocorneal endothelial syndrome

Clinical characteristics	ICE syndrome	Posterior polymorphous dystrophy	Axenfeld–Reiger's syndrome	Fuchs' dystrophy
Age of onset	Young/middle aged	Congenital or early childhood	Congenital	Middle aged to elderly
Laterality	Unilateral	Bilateral	Bilateral	Bilateral
Corneal abnormalities	Yes	Yes	No	Yes
Glaucoma	90%	25%	60%	5%
Iris atrophy	Yes	No	Yes	No
Iris nodules	Yes	No	No	No
Inheritance	No	Autosomal dominant	Autosomal dominant	No

abnormal endothelium and its abnormal basement membrane extend over the drainage angle and onto the iris.

The aetiology of these changes is not known, although a number of theoretical causes have been proposed. The most recently proposed is herpes simplex virus infection but this remains unconfirmed.

Diagnosis

ICE syndrome must be distinguished from other causes of stromal oedema and iris abnormalities, including Fuchs' endothelial dystrophy, Axenfeld–Reiger's anomaly and posterior polymorphous dystrophy, ischaemic iris atrophy, aniridia, iridoschisis, peripheral anterior synechiae from trauma or uveitis, angle abnormalities from neovascular glaucoma and uveitis, and iris nodules from neoplasia or neurofibromatosis. ICE syndrome can be distinguished from these similar entities on clinical grounds. Fuchs' dystrophy, posterior polymorphous dystrophy, and Axenfeld–Reiger's anomaly are those most commonly confused with ICE syndrome.

Treatment

Treatment of ICE syndrome is aimed at reducing the intraocular pressure to normal and overcoming corneal oedema. If the IOP is not raised and the cornea is normal or only mildly oedematous, as is often the case, no treatment is indicated. Elevated IOP should be managed medically in the first instance; restoring it to normal levels will often eliminate the corneal oedema. If the IOP cannot be managed medically, surgery may be necessary. If corneal oedema persists despite normal pressure and is symptomatic and troublesome, penetrating corneal transplantation is indicated.

Further reading

Akiya S, Takahashi H, Nakano N *et al.* Granular-lattice (Avellino) corneal dystrophy. *Ophthalmologica A* 1999; **213**: 58–62.

Akiya S, Brown SI. Granular dystrophy of the cornea. *Arch Ophthalmol* 1970; **84**: 179.

Akova YA, Kirkness CM, McCartney AC *et al.* Recurrent macular corneal dystrophy following penetrating keratoplasty. *Eye* 1990; **4**: 698.

Bron AJ, Brown NA. Some superficial corneal disorders. *Trans Ophthalmol Soc UK* 1971; **91**: 13.

Bron AJ, Burgess SEP. Inherited recurrent corneal erosion. *Trans Ophthalmol Soc UK* 1981; **101**: 239–43.

Brown NA, Bron AJ. Recurrent erosion of the cornea. *Br J Ophthalmol* 1976; **60**: 84.

Chandler PA. Atrophy of the stroma of the iris, endothelial dystrophy, corneal edema, and glaucoma. *Trans Am Ophthalmol Soc* 1955; **53**: 75.

Cibis JW, Krachmer JH, Phelps CD, Weingeist TA. The clinical spectrum of posterior polymorphous dystrophy. *Arch Ophthalmol* 1977; **95**: 1529.

Cogan DG, Reece AB. A syndrome of the iris nodules, ectopic Descemet's membrane and unilateral glaucoma. *Doc Ophthalmol* 1969; **26**: 424.

Eiburg H, Moller HU, Berendt I *et al.* Assignment of granular corneal dystrophy Groenoew type I (CDCG1) to chromosome 5q. *Eur J Hum Genet* 1994; **2**: 132–8.

Fine BS, Yanoff M, Pitts E, Slaughter FD. Meesmann's epithelial dystrophy of the cornea. *Am J Ophthalmol* 1977; **83**: 633.

Folberg R, Stone EM, Sheffield VC, Mathers WD. The relationship between granular, lattice type 1, and Avellino corneal dystrophies – a histopathologic study. *Arch Ophthalmol* 1994; **112**: 1080.

Fuchs A. Über primäre qeurtelfoermige Hornhauttrübung. *Klin Monatsbl Augenheilkd* 1939; **103**: 300.

Fujiki K, Kato T, Hotta Y *et al.* Seven different mutations detected in the BIGH3 (Kerato-epithelin) gene in Japanese corneal dystrophies (ARVO abstract 1762). *Invest Ophthalmol Vis Sci* 1999; **40** (suppl): S332.

Hall P. Reis–Bückler's dystrophy. *Arch Ophthalmol* 1974; **91**: 170.

Holland EJ, Daya SM, Stone EM *et al.* Avellino corneal dystrophy: clinical manifestations and natural history. *Ophthalmology* 1992; **99**: 1564.

Klintworth GK. Lattice corneal dystrophy: an inherited variety of amyloidosis restricted to the cornea. *Am J Pathol* 1967; **50**: 371.

Klintworth GK. Perspective. Advances in the molecular genetics of corneal dystrophies. *Am J Ophthalmol* 1999; **128**: 747–54.

Korvatska E, Munier FL, Djemai A *et al.* Mutation hot spots in 5q31-linked corneal dystrophies. *Am J Hum Genet* 1998; **62**: 320–4.

Kuwabara T, Cicarelli EC. Meesmann's corneal dystrophy. A pathological study. *Arch Ophthalmol* 1964; **71**: 676–82.

Levy SG, Kirkness CM, Ficker L, McCartney ACE. The histopathology of the iridocorneal-endothelial syndrome. *Cornea* 1996; **15**: 46.

Robin AL, Green WR, Lapsa TP *et al.* Recurrence of macular corneal dystrophy after lamellar keratoplasty. *Am J Ophthalmol* 1977; **85**: 457.

Small KW, Mullen L, Barletta J *et al.* Mapping of Reis–Bückler's corneal dystrophy to chromosome 5q. *Am J Ophthalmol* 1996; **121**: 384–90.

Stewart HS, Ridgway AE, Dixon MJ *et al.* Heterogeneity in granular corneal dystrophy: identification of three causative mutations in the TGFBI (BIGH3) gene – lessons for corneal amyloidogenesis. *Human Mutat* 1999; **14**: 126–32.

12 Corneal transplantation

A comprehensive discussion of corneal surgery is beyond the scope of this book but corneal transplantation is an important treatment for many corneal diseases fundamental to many aspects of clinical corneal disease, so it deserves consideration. Furthermore, the behaviour of corneal transplants demonstrates many important aspects of corneal biology.

Corneal transplantation was first proposed as a potential treatment for Egyptian ophthalmia in the first systematic textbook of medicine, published in 1797. The first lamellar graft was done by von Hippel in 1888 and the first penetrating graft by Zirm in 1906. Since then, the role of corneal transplantation has grown steadily and the procedure is practised more widely than all other forms of clinical allotransplantation combined. With corneal disease second only to cataract as a cause of blindness worldwide, corneal transplantation has the potential to reverse visual loss in millions of people. Unfortunately, the potential of the procedure is limited in two ways. First, by a shortage of corneas, particularly in places where corneal disease is common, such as in many rural communities in developing countries. Second, by allograft rejection, which is the major cause of graft failure and a particular problem in patients with acquired corneal disease following inflammatory disorders, the largest group of patients blinded by corneal disease.

The normal cornea is considered an immunologically privileged site. Patients with non-inflamed corneas and who have not had inflammation in the past, as is often the case with patients requiring corneal transplantation for dystrophies and keratoconus, are seldom troubled by corneal allograft rejection. However, for those who have an inflamed cornea and receive a corneal graft, as is sometimes necessary with infection and corneal perforation, allograft rejection occurs commonly, more commonly than it does in patients who have received kidney grafts or heart grafts. Inflammation erodes corneal privilege, even if the inflammatory episode occurred many years previous to the graft.

Transplantation biology

A normal cornea grafted into a normal recipient cornea is unlikely to reject; this can be considered to be the case with patients having grafts for keratoconus. Corneal privilege has been recognised for many years, for as long as allograft rejection has been appreciated, but the complicated origins of the phenomenon are only beginning to be understood. A number of mechanisms contribute, including the lack of blood vessels, antigen presenting cells and draining lymphatics in the normal cornea, and the constitutive expression of Fas ligand in the cornea which can induce apoptosis in invading lymphocytes and other bone marrow derived cells that find their way into the cornea to play an important role in the corneal allograft response.

Minor as well as major histocompatibility antigens are important in initiating a corneal allograft reaction. For this reason, as well as logistic reasons, conventional histocompatibility matching is of limited value in corneal transplantation.

There are other important differences between the mechanisms of corneal allograft rejection and the analogous process in other organs. Of particular note is that antigen presentation in the cornea is by the indirect route. Recipient antigen presenting cells, principally interstitial dendritic cells, present donor antigen to the host immunocytes. This is different from what occurs in the grafts of *vascularised* organs, such as kidney and liver, where donor passenger cells carried in the grafted vascular compartment present donor antigen to host immunocytes. This has some practical implications. Indirect presentation is MHC class II restricted, so that partial matching for class II antigens may be expected to worsen the outlook for corneal transplantation in someone prone to rejection; there is some evidence to support this.

Another consideration is that some part of the sensitisation to alloantigens in the cornea occurs remotely in the draining lymph nodes. A practical consequence of this is that topically delivered immunosuppressants, such as cyclosporin, which can be delivered as eye drops are not effective because they do not reach the lymph node where the effect takes place. Topical anti-inflammatory agents such as corticosteroids can be given topically but immunosuppressants cannot.

Once established, the corneal allograft reaction is directed against all cells in the donor cornea. It is, however, the damage inflicted by the process against the endothelium that is critical. The endothelium has limited capacity for repair and achieves a degree of restored function by the cells sliding and enlarging to cover any cell loss. There is little, if any, capacity for cell division. A full blown corneal allograft reaction may damage the endothelium irreparably, resulting in chronic oedema with blinding sequelae.

It is inflammation that erodes corneal privilege and threatens successful corneal transplantation. For successful transplantation, particularly in high risk cases, inflammation must be controlled and the consequences abrogated.

Indications for corneal transplantation

Corneal transplantation is done to overcome abnormalities in shape in otherwise virtually normal corneas, as in patients with keratoconus; to replace corneal opacities with normal transparent cornea, as is done for patients with scars or dystrophic deposits; to repair perforations or threatened perforations; and to replace non-functional endothelium that has resulted in corneal oedema. Keratoconus is the most common indication for corneal transplantation. Bullous keratopathy due to the trauma of cataract surgery or Fuchs' dystrophy is the next most common group. Because many grafts done in patients with inflammatory disorders of the cornea fail and need to be redone, regrafting in an eye with a previous failed graft is also common. The indications for corneal transplantation in Australia, as identified in the Australian Corneal Graft Registry, are set out in Box 12.1.

Preoperative assessment

It is important to be clear about the indication for corneal transplantation, to achieve shared expectations between patient and surgeon and for the patient to be made fully aware of the possible benefits and the risks to which they are exposed.

Generally speaking, for a patient to benefit visually from a corneal graft the vision achieved in the grafted eye must be equal to, or better than, the other eye. To be an unqualified success,

---

Box 12.1 *Indications for corneal transplantation in Australia (Australian Corneal Graft Registry Report 1996)*

Keratoconus	30%
Bullous keratopathy	25%
Failed previous graft	19%
Corneal dystrophy	7%
Scars and opacities	6%
Herpetic eye disease	5%
Other	8%

the operated eye must become the better of the two eyes. This is unlikely to be achievable in patients with unilateral postinflammatory scarring when the other eye has normal vision, so the risk of allograft rejection is so high in these cases that they are best left undone. Such patients have little to gain and are likely to be worse off when rejection occurs.

For some patients, corneal transplantation is undertaken to overcome the pain of bullous keratopathy. Many of these patients have had unsuccessful cataract surgery and have seriously disrupted eyes and limited visual potential. It is important that these patients understand that the operation is being done to overcome pain and that a good visual result should be considered a bonus.

Similarly, for patients requiring a corneal graft for corneal perforation or threatened perforation the aim is to preserve the integrity of the eye; good vision cannot be expected in the long term. Some additional surgery is likely to be necessary and patients must understand the limited prognosis.

The central consideration in the evaluation of the preoperative assessment is the balance of potential benefits and risks.

To assess this, it is necessary for the surgeon to estimate the risk of graft failure prior to surgery. This is important so that the patient can be warned of the risks to which they are exposed but also because it may be necessary to take additional measures to reduce the risk of allograft rejection and subsequent graft failure.

Risk comprises the probability of a problem occurring and the consequence of the problem should it arise. In the context of corneal transplantation, this means the surgeon must evaluate the risk of allograft rejection and the likely impact of graft failure. The risk of rejection can be estimated from the clinical signs of inflammation and the sequelae of inflammation. The presence of corneal vessels, active inflammation or history of inflammation in the past, previous graft failure, a raised IOP or history of elevated pressure in the past, or evidence of any previous intraocular

surgery on the eye, particularly of a previous corneal graft, are associated with an increased risk of rejection (Box 12.2).

The consequences of allograft rejection and graft failure are not trivial. At the very least, the chances of achieving success with a subsequent graft are substantially reduced. There is also considerable inconvenience and perhaps pain and discomfort as a consequence of corneal graft failure. There is no place for a "trial of corneal grafting" without being prepared to do all that is required to bring about success. Corneal graft failure should be avoided wherever possible.

Having evaluated the risk of failure, the next step for the surgeon and the patient is to weigh this against the potential benefits of the procedure. At one end of a spectrum are patients with keratoconus and at the other those with bilateral blindness due to postinflammatory scarring. With the latter group, there is much to be gained by the restoration of vision to one eye. This is enough to take a person from blindness to normal vision. To achieve this, however, there is the need for systemic immunosuppression with all its associated risks. For many patients, accepting the risk under these circumstances is justified. The risk cannot be justified if vision in the other eye is normal or if there has already been a successful graft in the first eye. With

---

Box 12.2 *Independent variables predicting failure of penetrating corneal grafts (Australian Corneal Graft Registry Report 1996)*

Surgeon identity
Corneal neovascularisation at the time of graft
History of inflammation in the grafted eye
Previous failed ipsilateral graft
Indication for graft other than keratoconus
Aphakia or pseudophakia
History of raised intraocular pressure
Neovascularisation of the graft
Occurrence of graft rejection episode
Microbial keratitis or stitch abscess in the graft
Early removal of graft sutures (<6 months postgraft)

keratoconus, the risk–benefit analysis is different because immunosuppression is not required. Under these circumstances, it is reasonable to recommend a transplant in the second eye; even though the functional benefits are limited, the risks encountered in pursuing these are minimal.

Patients for whom the risk of systemic immunosuppression can be justified must be carefully evaluated and advised. All patients taking effective doses of immunosuppressants experience untoward reactions, if not frank side effects. As much immunosuppression is required for patients receiving corneal transplantation in a high risk situation as is required to maintain a renal or liver graft. For this reason, this aspect of care is best managed by a physician working in solid organ transplantation.

Surgical principles

There are two principal aims in corneal transplantation surgery. First, to restore the transparency and curvature of the normal cornea and second, to minimise inflammation at all times. To achieve an appropriate curvature demands meticulous microsurgical technique; even in the best hands, post-transplantation astigmatism due to irregularities of corneal shape is a common outcome. To minimise inflammation also demands rigorous attention to surgical technique so as to minimise trauma, careful use of anti-inflammatory medication and close post-operative supervision to reduce the impact of postoperative inflammation from whatever cause.

Meticulous surgical technique implies excising a circular disc of cornea, replacing it with a donor cornea cut to precisely the same shape and suturing the graft in place so as to provide the appropriate curve for the transplanted cornea. All of this can be achieved with a very simple approach. Many complicated techniques have been developed and advocated, many of which require expensive equipment. Fortunately, none of this is required to do a meticulous job. The technique described below is simple and employs commonly used surgical instruments.

Surgical technique for corneal transplantation

1. Posture the eye; superior and inferior rectus suture (Figure 12.1).

2. Crossover suture with 6/0 silk on a spatulated needle, to hold the donor button in place at a later stage when the initial nylon sutures are to be used (Figure 12.2).

3. Paracentesis; for access to the anterior chamber without going through the wound (Figure 12.3).

4. Measure the size of the graft required. Do this by making a faint mark with a trephine of the most likely size, usually 7.5 mm.

5. Cut the donor button by placing it epithelium down on a firm plastic support and punching with a disposable trephine. The trephine should be larger than the planned recipient excision. Oversizing of 0.25 mm is appropriate for phakic cases and 0.5 mm for aphakic cases.

6. Cut the host cornea. Grasp the eye at the limbus with forceps, centre the trephine so that it can be observed axially with the microscope, being careful to ensure that the disc to be excised encloses the pathology to be resected. Cut the cornea by making smooth back and forth rotations of the trephine around its axis while applying firm even pressure. The cut made by the trephine should be deep but it is preferable not to penetrate the cornea at this stage (Figure 12.4). The wound is then deepened with a blade (Figure 12.5) and the cornea is penetrated in a controlled manner at a convenient point to introduce the corneal scissors (Figure 12.6). The scissors are introduced and excision of the disc is completed.

7. The donor disc is lifted into the defect in the recipient cornea (Figure 12.7) and 10/0 filament nylon is used to anchor the graft with four stitches at 6, 12, 9, and 3 o'clock.

These sutures must be carefully placed to ensure that the donor cornea is evenly distributed in the donor defect (Figure 12.8).

8. Definitive suturing. Either a continuous suture or 16 interrupted sutures of 10/0 nylon are used to fix the graft to the host cornea. A continuous suture is used if there is no focal pathology and the wound is likely to heal evenly. If, however, there are areas of scarring with vascularisation, uneven wound healing can be anticipated and it may be necessary to remove sutures from one part of the wound earlier than from other sections and it is therefore better to place interrupted sutures.

9. The continuous suture is tightened and the anterior chamber inflated with balanced salt solution (Figure 12.9).

Variations on basic surgical technique

If the patient is a child or aphakic or pseudo-phakic, it is necessary to support the globe so that it does not collapse when the eye is opened. This is done by sewing on a corneoscleral support ring at the beginning of the procedure (Figure 12.10).

Removal of a cataract is sometimes necessary at the time of corneal transplantation. This is achieved by curving a circular capsulorhexis and then adding four backcuts to facilitate expression of the nucleus. Aspiration of the cortex is more difficult in this situation with the eye open and some patience is required to ensure that removal of the cortex is achieved without engaging the capsule. Insertion of an intraocular lens is then relatively easy. A PMMA lens is preferred, the rigidity being useful in ensuring vitreous does not push the intraocular lens forward.

When dealing with aphakic eyes, it is sometimes necessary to remove vitreous from the anterior chamber and pupil. This is best done with a vitreous cutter but can be achieved with microsponges and scissors.

Surgical complications

Untoward events can occur during the surgery or at any time afterwards, even years or decades later.

Bleeding

At the time of operation, the most devastating complication is haemorrhage, particularly choroidal haemorrhage which may occur with any intraocular procedure where the IOP is suddenly reduced to atmospheric pressure and fragile choroidal vasculature ruptures. There is little that the surgeon can do in this situation other than close the eye as quickly as possible so as to restore the IOP and tamponade the bleeding. Haemorrhage can also occur from iris vessels and synechiae or even from corneal vessels. Bleeding from these origins is easier to manage and time alone will usually overcome the problem.

Damage to underlying structures

The iris and the lens can be damaged while excising the disc of the recipient cornea. The trephine may damage the underlying iris, causing a fixed dilated pupil postoperatively. Such a pupil is referred to as a Uritz–Savellia pupil and is a permanent but fortunately rare complication. Incision of the lens or iris occurs more frequently but is also rare.

Suture complications

A common complication is inclusion of the iris in the corneal stitches. Wherever possible, this should be rectified because postoperative synechiae predispose to corneal allograft rejection. Inaccurate suturing causing irregular forces to distort the cornea from its optimal shape is a common cause of postgraft astigmatism.

Postoperative complications

Complications manifesting after the surgical procedure is completed are related to aberrations in the biology of the graft and supporting host cornea.

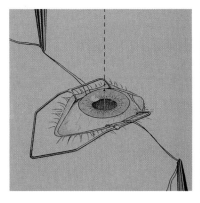

Figure 12.1 Posturing the eye. The optical system of the eye and the microscope are coaxial. This is achieved by carefully positioning the head and the use of superior and inferior rectus sutures

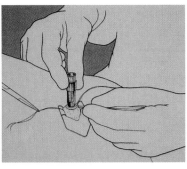

Figure 12.4 Trephination. The eye, trephine, and operating microscope are coaxial. Trephination is aimed at the same partial penetration at all points

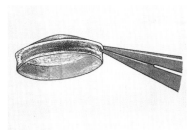

Figure 12.7 The donor disc is lifted from the punching block and placed into the recipient defect. Care is taken to grasp the epithelial rather than the endothelial edge

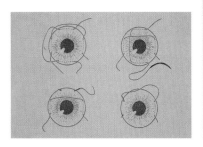

Figure 12.2 Crossover sutures of 6.0 silk on a spatulated needle are preplaced. These are used to assist stabilisation of the graft during the early suturing phase and as insurance against a sudden increase in intraocular pressure

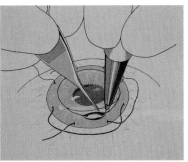

Figure 12.5 Deepening the trephination mark with a blade. The inner edge (i.e. the excised button) is grasped with forceps and the blade used to cut away for a small distance from the fixation point. The wound is then regrasped and another small advancement of the blade made

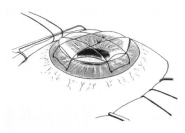

Figure 12.8 The donor is secured in the recipient defect by tying the crossover sutures and placing four cardinal sutures at 12, 3, 6, and 9 o'clock

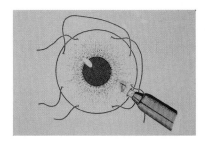

Figure 12.3 A paracentesis is made in an easily accessible meridian, for example adjacent to one of the crossover sutures

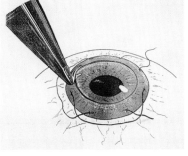

Figure 12.6 Final excision of recipient cornea with scissors. Curved corneal scissors are used to remove any remnants of attachment

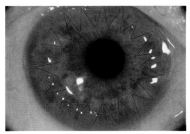

Figure 12.9 Continuous suture in a patient with keratoconus

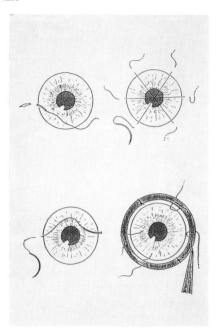

Figure 12.10 Corneoscleral support band. Three double-armed 6.0 silk sutures are preplaced, a flat metal band is placed over the sutures which are cut and tied to fixate the ring at six points

Primary graft failure

Primary graft failure occurs because the endothelium of the graft is not functioning. This may occur for a number of reasons related to the cause of death of the donor, the state of the donor eye, the way it was collected or the way in which or the length of time for which it was stored. If a graft does not clear within the first 10 days it should be replaced with another graft.

Corneal allograft rejection

This can occur at any time after transplantation. Immediate rejection such as can occur with solid organ transplants, where it is termed hyperacute rejection, seldom occurs in corneal transplantation. Corneal allograft rejection tends to occur later, as the wound is healing or after the donor cornea is populated with recipient cells. Rejection often complicates intercurrent inflammatory episodes, such as conjunctivitis, blepharitis, or keratitis. It manifests as an increase in ocular inflammation with increasing corneal oedema. Sometimes there is a linear accumulation of leucocytes on the endothelium; this arrangement is known as a *Khodadoust line*. At other times, there are keratic precipitates but without a linear arrangement (Figure 12.11).

Topical corticosteroids are the principal plank of therapy. Corticosteroids are given hourly for a few days. Then, as the process reverses, usually beginning within three or four days, the frequency can be reduced. In recalcitrant cases, oral steroids should also be given. When this is necessary, the course should not exceed 21 days and it is usual to give prednisolone 1 mg/kg/day for the first week and then reduce the dose to nothing over three weeks.

Astigmatism

Astigmatism is almost invariable after corneal transplantation and patients must be warned about the possibility. Astigmatism caused by irregular suture tension will disappear once the sutures are removed. It is only "sutures out" astigmatism that needs to be seriously considered. The aim should be to get the regular element of the astigmatism down to less than 5 dioptres, a level that can usually be managed

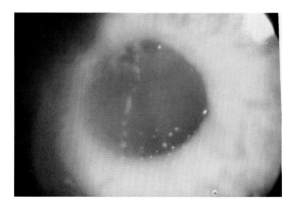

Figure 12.11 Corneal allograft rejection. Anterior segment inflammation with corneal oedema and a linear accumulation of leucocytes on the endothelium

with glasses or contact lenses. Higher levels can usually be reduced with simple incisional surgery, making accurate cuts in the graft margin in the steepest meridian. This can often be done under local anaesthesia at the slit lamp.

Astigmatism usually manifests soon after surgery or immediately after the sutures are removed. Dealing with the refractive correction in the year after the sutures are removed, that is in the second year after the graft, is the key element in achieving satisfactory visual outcomes after corneal transplantation.

Less commonly, astigmatism can occur decades after a successful corneal graft. This usually occurs in patients who have had surgery for keratoconus, in which case the ectatic process tends to begin centrally but with the passing years involves the peripheral cornea. As this occurs, the graft interface may become attenuated, resulting in wound stretch at one point or another; the central cornea tends to flatten in the meridian in which the stretching has occurred. Incisional surgery will not correct this type of postgraft astigmatism. Instead, the weakened wound must be strengthened by excision and suturing.

Infection

Infection can result from the use of contaminated donor material. With contemporary eye banking practices, this is a rare event. Delayed infection is more common and occurs in around 2% of cases. This is perhaps not surprising. Patients with corneal transplants have a foreign body in the cornea, the suture, and are receiving topical or even systemic immunosuppression. Infections around the suture tract are relatively common and although they are often caused by mildly pathogenic organisms susceptible to antimicrobial agents, poor outcomes are common. Allograft rejection and graft failure often complicate infections of this nature. Prompt recognition of the inflammatory process, identification of the causative organism,

and institution of appropriate antimicrobial chemotherapy are required if infected grafts are to be saved.

The range of organisms responsible for infecting corneal grafts reflects the commensal organisms of the external eye. Prolonged exposure to topical antibiotics and corticosteroids favours organisms of low pathogenicity, such as the nutritionally deficient streptococci and similar organisms causing infectious crystalline keratopathy (Figure 12.12). With this condition, chains of micro-organisms become visible in the cornea and there is little, if any, cellular response to the infection so that the organisms are seen to resemble crystals in the cornea.

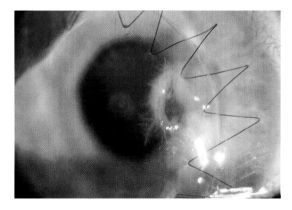

Figure 12.12 Infectious crystalline keratopathy in a patient with a corneal graft

Postoperative care

Great differences in outcome occur between centres, even when the case mix is similar. More than anything else, this reflects differences in postoperative management. Fastidious attention to detail over a prolonged postoperative period of years and meticulous attention to refractive requirements are necessary to achieve the full potential for patients. This can only be done with regular routine visits.

At our centre, patients who have corneal grafts are seen on day one after surgery, day seven, and then at three weeks, six weeks and 12 weeks, and then every three months after that until the suture is removed, which is typically after 12 months. At these visits, the graft is inspected, the IOP measured, and keratometry performed. At the slit lamp examination, particular attention is paid to the state of the epithelium, the presence of any inflammation, and the development of any new vessels in the vicinity of the graft margin.

Following removal of the suture, the frequency of the visits needs to be increased temporarily in order to ensure that patients are provided with the optimal refractive care. Because it is difficult to be sure of the integrity of the wound after the removal of sutures, patients should be seen a few days later and then six weeks after that. The graft shape tends to alter during the first six weeks after suture removal. When the shape is stable refraction should be carried out. Approximately 60% of patients with corneal grafts will need spectacles to achieve their required level of vision. Failure of spectacles to deliver this level of vision may be due to irregular corneal astigmatism due to warpage in the graft, excessive levels of regular astigmatism, usually beyond 5 dioptres or, less commonly, to anisometropia. Irregular astigmatism can only be dealt with by prescribing contact lenses. Excessive regular astigmatism can usually be overcome with simple incisional surgery. Anisometropia may require laser refractive surgery to reduce myopia.

Further reading

Aggarwal R. Deep lamellar keratoplasty: an alternative for penetrating keratoplasty (editorial). *Br J Ophthalmol* 1997; **81**: 178–9.

Aquavella JV, Van Horn DL, Haggerty CJ. Corneal preservation using M-K medium. *Am J Ophthalmol* 1975; **80**: 791.

Bourne WM. Corneal preservation: past, present, and future. *Refract Corneal Surg* 1991; 7: 60.

Castroviejo R. Keratoplasty. Comments on the technique of corneal transplantation. *Am J Ophthalmol* 1941; **24**: 1–20.

Coster DJ. Mechanisms of corneal graft failure: the erosion of corneal privilege. *Eye* 1989; **2**: 251–62.

Culbertson WM, Abbot RL, Froster RK. Endothelial cell loss in penetrating keratoplasty. *Ophthalmology* 1982; **89**: 600–4.

Doughman DJ. Prolonged donor preservation in organ culture: long term clinical evaluation. *Trans Am Ophthalmol Soc* 1980; **78**: 567–628.

Driebe WT, Stern GA. Microbial keratitis following corneal transplantation. *Cornea* 1983; **2**: 41.

Eisner G. *Eye Surgery*. New York: Springer-Verlag, 1980.

Filatov VP. Transplantation of the cornea. *Arch Ophthalmol* 1935; **13**: 321–47.

Hill JC. Systemic cyclosporin in high-risk keratoplasty: short versus long-term therapy. *Ophthalmology* 1994; **101**: 128–33.

Hiss JC, Maske R, Watson P. Corticosteroids in corneal graft rejection. Oral versus single pulse therapy. *Ophthalmology* 1991; **98**: 329.

Lindstrom RL. Advances in corneal preservation. *Trans Am Ophthalmol Soc* 1990; **88**: 555.

Lindstrom RL, Kaufman HE, Skelnik DL *et al.* Optisol corneal storage medium. *Am J Ophthalmol* 1992; **114**: 345.

O'Day DM. Diseases potentially transmitted through corneal transplantation. *Ophthalmology* 1989; **96**: 1133.

Pineros O, Cohen EJ, Rapuano CJ, Laibson PR. Longterm results after penetrating keratoplasty for Fuchs' endothelial dystrophy. *Arch Ophthalmol* 1996; **114**: 15–18.

Pineros O, Cohen EJ, Rapuano CJ, Laibson PR. Triple vs nonsimultaneous procedures in Fuchs' dystrophy and cataract. *Arch Ophthalmol* 1996; **114**: 525–8.

Urrets-Zavalia A. Fixed, dilated pupil, iris atrophy, and secondary glaucoma. A distinct clinical entity following penetrating keratoplasty in keratoconus. *Am J Ophthalmol* 1963; **56**: 257.

Volker-Dieben HJM. The effect of immunological and non-immunological factors on corneal graft survival. A single center study. *Doc Ophthalmol* 1982; **57**: 1–153.

Volker-Dieben HJ, D'Amaro J, Kok-van Alphen CC. Hierarchy of prognostic factors for corneal allograft survival. *Aust NZ J Ophthalmol* 1987; **15**: 11–18.

Williams KA, Muehlberg SM, Lewis RF, Coster DJ. How successful is corneal transplantation? A report from the Australian Corneal Graft Register. *Eye* 1995; **9**: 219–27.

Williams KA, Roder D, Esterman A *et al.* Factors predictive of corneal graft survival. Report from the Australian Corneal Graft Registry. *Ophthalmology* 1992; **99**: 403.

Zirm E. Eine erfolgreiche totale Keratoplastik. *Archiv für Ophthalmol* 1906; **64**: 580.

13 Medical therapy for corneal disease

Pharmacokinetics of drug delivery

The cornea is well situated for drug therapy. Because it is exposed on the surface of the eye, surrounded by the conjunctival sac and bathed in the tear film, drugs can be delivered directly to the site of corneal pathology. Therapeutic substances are absorbed directly into the cornea from the tear film and the conjunctival sac acts as a reservoir to ensure steady uptake of a drug over a period of time.

The normal cornea offers a significant barrier to drug absorption. Surface corneal epithelial cells have tight junctions, so that drugs must pass through the normal epithelial cells. Since they reach the epithelial cell through the tear film, solubility in lipid and water is required for optimal corneal absorption.

When the cornea is inflamed, the situation is different. The tight junctions between surface epithelial cells are compromised; gaps appear between the cells and absorption is facilitated. Some drugs have a similar effect; for example, benzylkonium chloride, commonly used as a preservative in eye drops, causes functional breaks in the epithelial membrane which facilitate drug absorption. Phenylephrine, another drug used topically, has a similar effect. Some factors influencing the absorption of drugs across the cornea are set out in Figure 13.1.

Routes of administration

Drug absorption into the cornea is excellent in most circumstances. Because higher drug levels can be achieved in corneal disorders such as inflammation and infection than can be achieved in the blood with systemic administration and because the chance of side effects is greatly reduced, topical administration of drugs to the cornea is almost always preferable to systemic administration. Topical preparations are also preferred to periocular injections; the drug levels achieved with topical medication are as high as can be achieved with subconjunctival or orbital injections and the high levels attained are more easily maintained. Topical administration is also less painful than periocular injections and more acceptable to patients. It must be remembered at all times that absorption through the cornea is sufficient to achieve blood levels in the pharmacological range and to create cross-reactions with other drugs the patient may be taking.

Drops or ointment?

Eye drops are preferable to ointments as they are more convenient to use. Ointments can interfere with vision and are largely impractical during the day. They also have a tendency to get under the healing epithelium to disturb vision and perhaps slow epithelial healing. This is another reason for avoiding ointments when treating corneal disease, particularly if there is an epithelial defect. However, some drugs, including the antiviral agents idoxuridine and acycloguanosine, can only be formulated in ointment form.

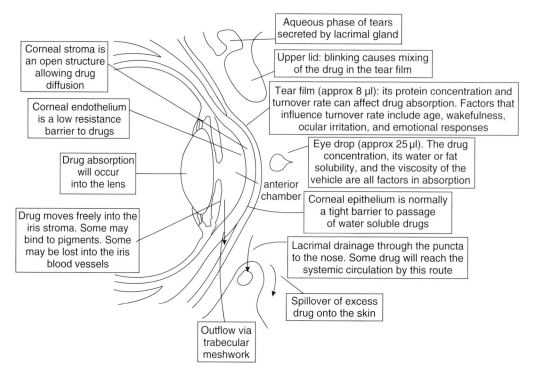

Figure 13.1   Some of the factors influencing the absorption of drugs by the eye

Besides the active agent, eye drops contain other chemicals, including buffers, stabilisers, and preservatives. It is necessary to look beyond the active agent when considering the use of a particular preparation.

Some drugs are not available commercially. This is usually the case with drugs offering no commercial opportunity for a drug company, either because the indication is rare, as is the case with anti-amoebic preparations, or because there is no patent protection of the drug use. Under these circumstances, it is necessary for ophthalmologists to have a pharmacy make up the preparation or to do it themselves.

Drugs used in the treatment of corneal diseases

A large number of drugs are used for the treatment of corneal diseases.

Diagnostic preparations

Dyes

Two related diagnostic dyes are commonly used, fluorescein and rose bengal. Both are used to examine the ocular surface and fluorescein is also used in applanation tonometry and contact lens fitting. For these purposes, both dyes are available as eye drops. They are also available impregnated into paper strips. The drops are preferred over the paper preparations.

When used for examining the ocular surface, one drop of the solution is instilled directly onto the cornea. The patient is asked to look down, the upper lid is retracted and a drop is put directly onto the superior cornea (Figure 13.2).

Although both dyes are used extensively, both have disadvantages. Fluorescein tends to stain the cornea and aqueous humour, making interpretation of other signs more difficult. Rose

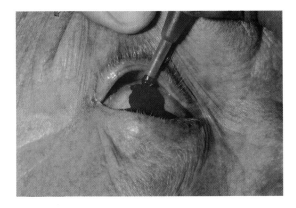

Figure 13.2 The administration of fluorescein and rose bengal prior to the slit lamp examination. The patient looks down, the upper lid is held up to expose the superior bulbar conjunctiva onto which a drop of the dye is applied

bengal can cause considerable discomfort so that a local anaesthetic agent is often used and this can also alter the signs. Nevertheless, these two dyes are important in all cornea and external disease clinics.

Fluorescein stains denuded basement membrane and stroma and is used extensively to identify corneal ulcers. However, it does not stain abnormal epithelium nearly as well as rose bengal and therefore has more limited uses. Because it is easily seen in the tear film and does not stain the corneal epithelium unless it is seriously abnormal, fluorescein is useful for applanation tonometry and contact lens fitting.

Rose bengal stains all epithelial cells unprotected by normal mucus coverage. It stains epithelial cells affected by tear film deficiency and abnormal or deficient differentiation. In cells affected by abnormal nutrition, as occurs in tear film disorders, toxic or dystrophic or neoplastic changes stain obviously, as does the epithelial edge of corneal ulcer.

Local anaesthetic agents

The cornea is richly supplied with sensory nerves so that minor corneal pathology can be painful. Instillation of a topical anaesthetic agent is often necessary to adequately examine the cornea. Patients with painful corneal conditions, such as corneal abrasions, receive instant relief from pain with one drop of local anaesthetic agent. All local anaesthetic agents are toxic and should only be used for diagnostic purposes and to carry out procedures on the eye, such as suture removal, micropuncture of epithelium, biopsies, and removal of lesions such as pterygia. They should not be used as therapeutic agents.

There are two groups of local anaesthetic agents and both are available as topical preparations for use in the eye. One group contains esters of derivatives of para-aminobenzoic acids, the other group are amides and derivatives of aniline. The commonly used anaesthetic agents are all members of one of these two groups.

Ester linkage:

- esters of benzoic acid, e.g. cocaine
- esters of meta-aminobenzoic acid, e.g. proparacaine
- Esters of para-aminobenzoic acid, e.g. procaine, chlorococaine, tetracaine, benoxinate.

Amide linkage (amides of benzoic acid):

- lidocaine
- mepivacaine
- bupivacaine
- etidocaine.

The cornea is readily anaesthetised, both by topical application of anaesthetic agents and by injection into the retrobulbar or subconjunctival space. Furthermore, all indications for local anaesthesia of the cornea for diagnosis or surgical procedures require only a relatively brief period of effect. For these reasons, only a limited number of the various agents available need to be considered for use. Lidocaine, as an injectable agent, and proparacaine hydrochloride, as a topical agent, are satisfactory for all circumstances.

Cycloplegics and mydriatics

These agents are used for diagnostic and therapeutic purposes. Often corneal disease is associated with a reactive miosis which contributes to a patient's discomfort. In this situation cycloplegia and mydriasis are beneficial in increasing comfort. Corneal disease is also associated with intraocular inflammation that may threaten the development of posterior synechiae and even pupil block. Mydriasis is also indicated in this situation.

Cycloplegic mydriatics are indicated for these conditions. These are anticholinergic agents which block cholinergic activation of the sphincter muscle of the iris, resulting in dilation of the pupil and the muscle of the ciliary body, leading to cycloplegia. The choices available to the clinician are atropine, homatropine, cyclopentolate, and tropicamide. A judgement is made as to the duration of treatment likely to be needed. If it is a week or more, atropine is indicated; the onset of action is slightly slower than for the other agents but the length of action is prolonged, so that all that is required is administration once a day, which is another advantage in using atropine in this circumstance. Patients with corneal and intraocular inflammation are often using a number of topical medications and are likely to incur problems with toxicity. The once daily administration of atropine imposes a lesser load on the cornea than the more frequent administration of the other alternatives.

If a shorter period of treatment is required, the other possibilities are homatropine or cyclopentolate, which can be given twice daily. An advantage of these drugs is that accommodation returns quickly when they are withdrawn.

Cycloplegics and mydriatics are used routinely in all eye clinics. They can alter the clinical signs of corneal disease. Therefore, for patients presenting with corneal disease, examination of the cornea must come before the instillation of any drops, including cycloplegics and mydriatics. These drugs will affect the corneal epithelium by creating widespread punctate epithelial erosions and if they contain phenylephrine, the vessels will constrict, giving a shortlived reduction in the inflammatory score.

Therapeutic agents

Anti-inflammatory agents

Corneal inflammation is common and threatening. Anti-inflammatory agents are frequently employed to treat corneal disease and the introduction of topical corticosteroid preparations in the 1960s was one of the most important advances in the treatment of inflammatory eye disease. Like all major advances, considerable controversy surrounded their introduction. They are powerful and effective medicine with the capacity to reduce the host response and thereby to make unsuspected infections worse. They were also believed to cause stromal melting. Thirty years later, their use is no longer controversial. Infections should not go unrecognised, but there is a much better understanding of the process of corneolysis and corticosteroids have been excused.

Corticosteroids have many distinct and measurable effects on inflammation within the cornea. One of the most important of these anti-inflammatory mechanisms is the inhibition of leucocyte migration into the cornea. Much of the corneal destruction which occurs with inflammation results from the degranulation of invading leucocytes and the release of lytic enzymes. Unquestionably, the accumulation of polymorphonucleocytes in an inflamed cornea can be reduced by the administration of topical steroids, if they are given early enough. Although not the only anti-inflammatory action of corticosteroids, the impairment of white cell recruitment into the cornea is used as a measure of anti-inflammatory activity of drugs. These bone marrow derived cells also have an important role in killing invading micro-organisms. A reduction in the population of white cells, or a functional impairment in those that are present, will tip the balance in favour of the micro-organism and worsen the impact of infection. Clearly, corticosteroids should be avoided if there is any possibility of undiagnosed infection.

Another complication of the use of topical corticosteroids is the development of raised IOP which occurs in up to 20% of patients. It is more of a problem for patients with anterior segment inflammation because drug absorption is greater, the intraocular levels achieved are higher, and perhaps because drainage mechanisms are compromised by the disease process. The tendency for some patients to develop raised IOP is an important limitation on the usefulness of topical corticosteroids for patients with corneal disease.

The anti-inflammatory activity of corticosteroids is related to the chemical structure of the steroid, the way in which it is prepared (water soluble salts, esters, or suspensions) and the concentration of the steroid preparation.

All other factors being equal, dexamethasone, betamethasone, and fluoromethalone are of comparable effectiveness with respect to the inhibition of white cell recruitment. In this, they are more effective than prednisolone, which is in turn more effective than hydrocortisone.

Acetate esters of a particular steroid have stronger anti-inflammatory activity at the same concentration. These preparations are suspensions rather than solutions and must be dispersed by shaking the bottle before use.

Toxicity from topical corticosteroids is often an issue when treating corneal disorders. Inflamed corneas are more prone to show the signs of drug toxicity than non-inflamed corneas. This is partly due to the increased absorption of the drug but is also related to the vulnerable state of the corneal epithelium. Another factor is the prolonged time over which patients need to be treated.

Acetate suspensions tend to be more toxic to the corneal epithelium than soluble salts. For this reason, the clinician is often required to use a phosphate salt preparation rather than a more active acetate suspension in order to minimise the risk of toxicity. In most situations, prednisolone phosphate 0.5% is an appropriate agent for treating inflammatory corneal disease. If the inflammation does not subside with this preparation, then a stronger but more toxic preparation, such as prednisolone acetate 1%, can be substituted.

Clinicians should develop a consistent approach to the use of topical corticosteroids. By using the one preparation most of the time, a clinician becomes familiar with the response to the drug. An informal comparison between what the clinician expects and what is observed in a particular case is useful in titrating medication against inflammatory score.

Non-steroidal anti-inflammatory agents

This group of drugs has been available to ophthalmologists for some time but they do not have an established place in the treatment of corneal disease. If a cornea is inflamed and needs treatment, corticosteroids remain the most effective option.

Antibacterial agents

There are two separate indications for the use of antibacterial agents in the treatment of corneal conditions: as prophylaxis when the epithelium has been breached and there is a risk of infection, and for the treatment of established bacterial infections.

Chloramphenicol

Prophylaxis demands a broad spectrum agent. Chloramphenicol has proved very effective in this situation because it has a broad spectrum and very little local toxicity or contact allergy. There is, however, a long-standing concern about the risk of topical chloramphenicol causing aplastic anaemia. There is no doubt that systemic chloramphenicol causes aplastic anaemia but there is doubt as to whether topical chloramphenicol does the same thing. A fear of local administration causing aplastic anaemia and a well developed desire to escape ubiquitous litigation mean that the use of chloramphenicol is avoided in the United States, although it is widely used elsewhere. In the United Kingdom and in Europe generally, and in Asia and Australia, chloramphenicol has been used extensively for many years where a broad spectrum antibiotic is required for prophylaxis.

Aminoglycosides and cephalosporins

Established infections demand highly specific therapy. For many years, topical cephalosporins, such as cephalothin, have been used to treat Gram positive infections and topical aminoglycosides, such as gentamicin, have been used to treat Gram negative infections. By and large, this has been a very successful approach. Some concern has been expressed about drug resistance but this has not proven to be a limiting factor, perhaps because the drug levels achieved by topical administration are so high that the usual concerns about reaching the minimal inhibitory concentration for a particular organism do not become an issue. Although the commercial preparations of aminoglycosides are probably adequate, many ophthalmologists prefer to prepare more concentrated drops. The cephalosporins have never been available commercially because they are unstable and tend to break down in days or weeks, so that a fresh preparation must be provided every 4–5 days. Because of these difficulties, broad spectrum oxyquinolones have been introduced into ophthalmic practice.

Fluroquinolones

These have a broad spectrum and are active against most of the bacteria causing corneal infections. Because they are stable, they can be made up commercially and because of the breadth of their activity, only one preparation need be employed to treat most corneal infections. In many parts of the world, this monotherapy approach has replaced the combined use of aminoglycosides and cephalosporins. Some ophthalmologists prefer to continue with dual therapy, which has worked very well over many years and has a broader spectrum than fluroquinolones used alone. Resistance of streptococci to fluroquinolones is a significant limitation. Furthermore, because the Gram stain predicts the causative organism 70% of the time, only one agent (either an aminoglycoside or cephalosporin) is required most of the time.

Antifungal agents

Antifungal agents are required to treat keratomycosis and endophthalmitis. The patterns of susceptibility of fungi are much less predictable than those of bacteria, so that treatment is more empirical. Antifungal agents fall into two broad classifications: the polyenes, such as natamycin, and the imidazoles, such as ketaconazole and miconazole. These have different modes of action and should be used together in most situations. A typical combination is miconazole 1% eye drops and natamycin 5% ointment. The natamycin can be obtained from Alcon on special request and the miconazole (or alternative imidazole preparation) needs to be made up by the ophthalmologist.

Anti-amoebic agents

Amoebic keratitis can be treated with several agents effective against acanthamoeba. The two most popular preparations are Brolene ointment and PHMB (polyhexaminemethaminebromide) drops. Both of these agents are effective, but care must be taken to avoid local toxicity, particularly with Brolene.

Acetyl cysteine

This acts as a mucolytic agent. It is widely used in respiratory medicine to break down mucus plugs in the pulmonary airways. When mucus secretion troubles the cornea, as it may do by causing filamentary keratitis in patients with dry eyes or shield ulcers in patients with severe atopic disease, one drop of a 10% solution each day is usually sufficient to break down adherent mucus.

Retinoic acid

This has a useful role in the treatment of squamous metaplasia, especially when the corneal epithelium has become keratinised. Retinoic acid can be prepared either as a drop or an ointment. The ointment preparation of all-trans retinoic acid administered once a day is often effective in reversing keratinisation of the ocular surface when all other approaches have failed.

Systemic anti-inflammatory therapy for corneal disease

Although topical steroids are the most effective treatment for corneal inflammation, it is occasionally necessary to use systemic therapy. The usual reason for this is that topical therapy has raised the IOP. Under these conditions two options are oral non-steroidal agents or systemic steroids.

Oral non-steroidal agents are not always effective, but there are fewer risks associated with their use than with systemic steroids. If there is time to try these agents as a first step, because the cornea is not acutely threatened, it is preferable to do so even if the chances of success are not high. If they do not control corneal inflammation, it is necessary to resort to systemic steroids. These are very effective at controlling corneal inflammation but are prone to cause serious side effects.

In an acute situation the usual starting dose is 1 mg/kg/day or about 75 mg a day. This dose is not sustainable in the long term but is usually effective in controlling the inflammation initially. The dose can usually be decreased quickly, halving it over each ensuing week. Oral steroids tend to be more effective at controlling inflammation initially than they are at maintaining control. Often, inflammation returns as the dose is reduced. This demands a low maintenance dose of steroids that will not produce unsatisfactory side effects, but such a dose will often not control the inflammation so that it is necessary to add a steroid sparing drug.

In some cases, such as with corneal allograft reaction and some autoimmune diseases, it may be possible to use cyclosporin for this.

Systemic immunosuppression for corneal disease

For some threatening conditions, systemic immunosuppression is indicated. The two most frequent indicators are for prevention of allograft rejection in high risk cases and for the treatment of destructive corneal diseases considered to have an immunological basis. Despite advances in this area of therapeutics, the side effects of immunosuppression can be serious and even life threatening.

Generally, the use of systemic immunosuppression is reserved for patients in whom successful treatment is required to avoid disability and blindness. Since the indications for systemic immunosuppression are rare, most ophthalmologists manage patients requiring this treatment themselves. This is best done with the help of physicians more experienced in the field.

No firm guidelines are available regarding the use of particular immunosuppressive agents for the treatment of corneal disorders. Steroids are particularly effective immunosuppressive agents but are relatively non-specific in their effects and are associated with serious side effects when administered systemically for any length of time. A steroid sparing approach is required for most patients. One approach is to combine three therapies: systemic corticosteroids, cyclosporin, and azathioprine. An initial high dose of

Table 13.1   Drugs used for systemic immunosuppression in patients with threatening corneal disorders

Drug	Oral dose	Adverse effects	Monitoring
Prednisolone	1 mg/kg/day morning dose	Cataracts, glaucoma, diabetes, hypertension, myopathy, osteoporosis, mood swings	Monthly: weight, blood pressure, blood glucose
Cyclosporin	5 mg/kg/day morning and evening doses	Renal toxicity Hypertension	Monthly: blood pressure, serum creatinine, serum electrolytes, liver function tests
Azathioprine	1–1.5 mg/kg/day	Nausea, flu-like symptoms, myelosuppression	Monthly: blood count, liver function tests

prednisolone (1 mg/kg/day) is followed by a rapidly declining dose so that it is no longer given after 21 days, but the cyclosporin and azathioprine are continued.

Patients receiving systemic immunosuppression require careful monitoring of their general health status and blood tests to monitor bone marrow and liver function. They need to be monitored at least monthly (Table 13.1).

Management of inflammatory disorders of the cornea

Many different conditions, such as infection, trauma, autoimmune conditions, and allograft reactions, are associated with inflammation in the cornea. Since acute inflammation or sustained chronic inflammation are threatening to vision, it is usually necessary to suppress inflammation even when there is a specific treatable cause such as infection. The management of inflammation is a fundamental aspect of management of corneal disease. Since the principles are the same whatever the underlying cause, it is important to consider them in some detail.

The amount of inflammatory medication given to patients with corneal inflammatory disease is titrated against the level of the inflammatory reaction in the cornea. This is necessary because all effective therapy comes at a price. The side effects of topical therapy can be considerable and exposure to such agents should be kept to a minimum. In order to titrate the dose of anti-inflammatory medication against the level of inflammatory reaction, it is necessary to be able to quantify both.

Corneal inflammatory score

Any attempt to quantify clinical signs is inevitably somewhat arbitrary. One scoring system used over the years involves giving a number to the various relevant clinical signs and adding them together to get the "corneal inflammatory score". A simple three-point scale is used for most of the signs and a binary system is used for others (Table 13.2).

Table 13.2 Qualification of corneal inflammatory signs to assist the titration of topical anti-inflammatory agents against corneal inflammation

Sign	Degree	Score
Bulbar injection	Mild	1
	Moderate	2
	Severe	3
Corneal epithelial oedema	Present	1
	Absent	0
Corneal stromal oedema	Absent	0
	Less than one quadrant	1
	One or two quadrants	2
	Three or four quadrants	3
Corneal stromal infiltrate	Absent	0
	Less than one quadrant	1
	One or two quadrants	2
	Three or four quadrants	3
Corneal stromal (active) vessels	Absent	0
	Single leash in one quadrant	1
	One or two quadrants	2
	Three or four quadrants	3
Intraocular pressure	Less than 20 mmHg	0
	More than 20 mmHg	1
Maximum total corneal inflammatory score		14

The hard numbers are useful, but the major benefit of this approach is the discipline required to measure inflammation objectively.

Anti-inflammatory potency of topical medication

There is considerable variation in the anti-inflammatory effect of the agents employed to treat corneal inflammation. Two broad classes of drugs are used: steroidal and non-steroidal anti-inflammatory agents. Currently, only the steroidal topical agents have found a place in the treatment of serious corneal inflammatory disease.

Factors influencing the effectiveness of topical steroids used for the treatment of corneal inflammation include the configuration of the active steroidal agent, the way it is formulated, and the concentration of the drug.

The anti-inflammatory activity of the steroids used in topical ophthalmic preparations is usually measured against the effect of hydrocortisone. If the anti-inflammatory activity of hydrocortisone is considered to be one unit, the activity of prednisolone is considered to be four and that of dexamethasone and betamethasone to be 16.

The absorption and therefore the bioavailability of the steroid are influenced by the way it is prepared. Acetates are insoluble in water but are prepared as suspensions; in this form, they are better absorbed and more potent in the cornea than phosphate salts that are soluble. The soluble preparations are, however, less toxic to the cornea when used for prolonged periods.

Not unexpectedly, the more concentrated the preparation, the greater the absorption. One percent preparations are more effective than 0.5% preparations of the same drug. Toxicity is also related to concentration as well as to the nature of the preparation.

Absorption of drugs across the cornea is increased if the cornea is altered from its normal state. With this increased absorption comes a greater therapeutic effect but increased side effects. The state of the cornea must be taken into account when prescribing drugs to treat corneal disease. The corneal epithelium is normally an effective barrier against the movement of drugs into the stroma and anterior chamber, but this barrier function is reduced when the cornea is inflamed and lost altogether when the epithelium has been lost. Chemical agents present in topical preparations can also influence the barrier function of the cornea. For example, thiomersol and benzylkonium chloride can open up the spaces between epithelial cells, increasing the uptake of concomitantly administered drugs.

Dose schedules: initial dose and titration

In most situations, prednisolone phosphate 0.5% given four times a day is an appropriate starting point. This is somewhere in the middle of the scale of effectiveness of commercially available preparations. It is sufficiently effective to control inflammation in most clinical situations but not likely to be toxic, at least in the intermediate term of 8–12 weeks. When patient is commenced on steroids, the inflammatory

Table 13.3 Topical preparations used to treat corneal disease. These are drops unless otherwise stated

	Commercial	Self-prepared
Antibacterial		
Cephalothin		50 mg/ml
Gentamicin	3 mg/ml	15 mg/ml
Ofloxacin	3 mg/ml	
Ciprafloxacin	3 mg/ml	
Penicillin G		5000 U/ml
Tobramycin	15 mg/ml	
Vancomycin	50 mg/ml	
Chloramphenicol	5 mg/ml	
Antifungal		
Amphotericin		3 mg/ml
Miconazole		1%
Natamycin	50 mg/ml	
Antiprotozoal		
Propamidine isothianate	0.1% (1 mg/ml)	
Polyhexamethylene biguanide		200 micrograms/ml
Dyes		
Fluorescein	1% single dose 2% single dose	
Bengal rose	1% single dose	
Topical anaesthetics		
Lignocaine	4%	
Proxymetacaine	0.5%	
Amethocaine	0.5% 1%	
Cycloplegics and mydriatics		
Homatropine	2%, 5%	
Atropine	0.5% 1%	
Cyclopentolate	0.5%, 1%	
Tropicamide	0.5%, 1%	
Phenylephrine	2.5%, 5%, 10%	
Anti-inflammatory agents		
Hydrocortisone – suspension	0.5%, 1%	
– ointment	0.5%,1%	
Prednisolone – phosphate	0.5%	
– acetate	0.5%	
Dexamethosone – phosphate	N/A	
– alcohol	0.1%	
Fluoromethalone– acetate	0.1%	
– suspension	0.1%	
Mucolytic		
Acetyl cysteine	10%	
Antimitotic agents		
Mitomycin C	0.02%	
Differentiation promoter		
Retinoic acid (ointment)	0.05%	

score is recorded; when the patient returns, the inflammatory signs are scored and compared with the initial score. If the score is the same or more, the frequency of administration can be increased; the preparation can be given as often as hourly. If this does not control the inflammation as judged quantitatively, then it is necessary to consider a more potent preparation, such as prednisolone acetate 1%. If, however, the inflammatory score is reduced, the dose of steroids can be reduced accordingly. Instead of using prednisolone four times a day, the frequency of administration can be reduced to three times a day. It is preferable not to reduce the frequency of steroid administration more often than every second week because this may lead to rebound inflammation which will require an increase in the dosage. It is better to allow the corneal inflammation to subside for a reasonable length of time, usually around two weeks at a time, in order to avoid inflammatory "rebound".

Side effects of topical corticosteroids

The two most troublesome side effects of topical steroids are raised IOP and the enhancement of some infections.

Many individuals will experience an increase of IOP when given topical steroids. It is mandatory that everyone receiving these agents has their intraocular pressure monitored regularly. The pressure raising effects of steroids vary with the dose and state of the epithelium. Generally, the more effective a preparation is at controlling inflammation, the more likely it is to increase inflammation. For this reason, it is desirable to use a preparation that will control the inflammation, but to avoid using preparations that are stronger than necessary for the particular clinical situation. Patients who are pressure responders and who have corneal inflammatory disease requiring treatment are in a particularly difficult situation. It is not always clear whether the elevated IOP is the result of corneal inflammation or a consequence of its treatment and in some cases the only way to resolve this is to withdraw the topical steroids and observe what happens to the IOP. If the raised

pressure is due to the steroids and the patient does need anti-inflammatory treatment, then the choices are limited. First, the dose can be reduced to the lowest that will control the inflammation and the pressure effect of this dose can be assessed. If the pressure remains too high, then it may be necessary to resort to systemic anti-inflammatory medications.

The second major complication of the use of topical steroids is the enhancement of unsuspected infections. Herpes simplex virus infection of the corneal epithelium is made worse by the use of topical steroids. Dendritic keratitis is made much worse and may turn into geographic ulceration with underlying stromal disease. Patients with interstitial keratitis who are misdiagnosed and treated with topical steroids without antiviral cover may develop severe corneal ulceration. Fungal infections are also made worse by the use of topical steroids. With bacterial infections, the picture is more complicated; some are made worse and some are not. Evidence from *in vivo* studies indicates that infection with Gram-positive bacteria is not influenced by the use of topical steroids, but that infection with Pseudomonas is made worse if topical steroids are used on their own. If they are used in combination with an effective antibiotic, the steroids do not influence the course of the infection although the number of polymorpholeucocytes recruited into the cornea is reduced.

The message for clinical practice is that if there is any chance that corneal inflammation is due to infection, topical steroids should not be used until the causative organism has been identified and even then, they should only be used with due caution. If it is suspected that herpes simplex virus is in the cornea, an antiviral agent should be used concomitantly.

Further reading

Fraunfelder FT. *Drug Induced Ocular Side Effects and Drug Interactions.* Philadelphia: Lea & Febiger, 1976.

Mishima S. Pharmacology of ophthalmic solutions. *Contact Intraocular Lens Med J* 1978; **4**: 22–46.

Raizman M. Corticosteroid therapy of eye disease. Fifty years later. *Arch Ophthalmol* 1996; **114**: 1000–1.

14 Procedures

At various points in the text reference has been made to procedures used in the diagnosis of corneal disease. A *brief* description of these procedures is set out in the following section. The indications, setting in which the procedure can be done, the equipment required, and the essential steps in the procedure are described along with the most commonly encountered complications and the desirable follow up.

- Amniotic membrane transplantation
- Botulinum toxin-A induced ptosis
- Conjunctival biopsy
- Conjunctival flap – Gunderson's
- Conjunctival flap – pedicle
- Corneal biopsy
- Corneal micropuncture
- Corneal scraping
- Corneal transplantation
- Corneal transplantation in an infant
- Corneal transplantation with lens extraction and intraocular lens insertion
- Gram stain
- Lavage of chemical burns
- Limbal transplantation
- Pedicled conjunctival flap to close corneal perforation
- Pterygium excision and conjunctival graft
- Removal of a calcified band keratopathy
- Tarsorrhaphy
- Tissue adhesive – corneal perforation

Amniotic membrane transplantation

Indications	1. In limbal stem cell deficiency amniotic membrane transplantation can be done in combination with stem cell graft. 2. Chemical injuries 3. Persistent epithelial defects 4. Painful bullous keratopathy 5. Conjunctival cicatrisation
Setting	Operating room
Equipment required	1. Speculum 2. Plain forceps 3. Conjunctival forceps 4. 10.0 nylon suture, 8.0 polyglactin 910 suture 5. Bandage contact lens
Anaesthesia	1. Topical 2. Regional – local infiltration, peribulbar, subtenon
Procedure	1. The amniotic membrane is gently spread on a prepared corneal surface and trimmed to the appropriate size 2. In corneal/limbal diseases the membrane should be larger than the area involved 3. Fix the amniotic membrane with 10.0 nylon and 8.0 polyglactin 910 on the cornea and conjunctival ends respectively 4. In conjunctival surgery, it is used to cover conjunctival defects, using a spacer to maintain fornices 5. A bandage contact lens is then placed for comfort and also to hold the graft
Complications	1. Operative – haemorrhage, perforation of globe 2. Postoperative – failed epithelialisation, fibrosis, infection
Follow up and postoperative care	1. The contact lens and sutures are removed after 2–4 weeks 2. Topical antibiotics and corticosteroids – preservative free are preferred

Botulinum toxin-A induced ptosis

Indications	1. Some persistent epithelial defect 2. Exposure keratopathy
Setting	Procedure room
Equipment required	1. Botulinum toxin-A (reconstituted with isotonic saline to the appropriate dilution) 62.5 picagrams in 0.1 ml 2. A 25 mm, 25 gauge needle or a tuberculin syringe
Anaesthesia	Local to skin or not required
Procedure	The skin is penetrated immediately below the central part of the superior orbital rim and the needle passed backwards along the orbital roof for 25 mm. The effect lasts for seven days to five weeks
Complications	1. Transient ipsilateral superior rectus palsy 2. Haemorrhage

Conjunctival biopsy

Indications	1. Suspected conjunctival malignancy 2. To establish a diagnosis of systemic diseases with conjunctival involvement, e.g. sarcoidosis 3. Early diagnosis of suspected autoimmune conjunctivitis
Setting	1. Procedure room with operating microscope 2. Operating room
Equipment required	1. Speculum 2. Conjunctival forceps (plain) 3. Conjunctival scissors
Anaesthesia	1. Topical 2. Regional – local infiltration, peribulbar, subtenon, subconjunctival
Procedure	1. Identify the site or sites for biopsy 2. A subconjunctival injection of 2% lignocaine 3. Gently dissect the lesion. Minimise handling the tissue as this can create artefacts 4. If the lesion is large multiple biopsies can be done 5. Each biopsy is placed in a separate bottle accompanied by a map
Managing the specimen	1. Histopathology – isotonic buffered formaldehyde 2. Immunohistochemical staining (autoimmune diseases) – direct immunofluorescence fixative
Follow up and postoperative care	1. Topical antibiotics, e.g. chloramphenicol until the conjunctiva heals

Conjunctival flap – Gunderson's

Indications	1. Corneal perforation which has failed to respond to other modalities of treatment and not suitable for keratoplasty 2. Corneal oedema (painful bullous keratopathy) 3. Chronic epithelial defects which have failed to respond to conventional medical therapy
Setting	1. Operating room
Equipment required	1. Speculum 5. Plain forceps 2. 4.0 silk suture 6. 6.0 polyglactin 910 suture 3. Bard Parker no. 15 blade 7. Needle holder 4. Conjunctival scissors
Anaesthesia	1. Regional – local infiltration with 1% lignocaine with epinephrine (1: 100 000) peribulbar, subtenon
Procedure	1. Place a superior rectus bridle suture 2. Once the local anaesthetic has been administered, the conjunctiva is cut 15–18 mm above the superior limbus for approx. 30 mm horizontally. Avoid tenons. Dissect inferiorly till the superior limbus 3. Next a 360° periotomy is performed 4. Prepare the corneal surface by removing the corneal epithelium and necrotic stroma, if present, by gentle scraping with a blade 5. The flap is now placed over the cornea and secured with 6.0 polyglactin 910 6. The original conjunctiva of the lower limbus is approximated to the lower border of the bridge flap, closed with two interrupted sutures. Repeat for the superior limbus
Complications	1. Operative – haemorrhage, button hole of the conjunctiva 2. Postoperative – retraction of the conjunctival flap infection
Follow up and postoperative care	1. Topical antibiotics and topical inflammatory treatment 2. The inflammation gradually settles after a few weeks and the flap continues to thin over several months 3. Review at one day, one week, then as required

Conjunctival flap – pedicle

Indications	1. Corneal perforation which has failed to respond to other modalities of treatment 2. Chronic epithelial defect which has failed to respond to conventional medical therapy
Setting	1. Operating room
Equipment required	1. Speculum 5. Plain forceps 2. 4.0 silk sutures 6. 10.0 nylon sutures 3. Bard Parker no. 15 blade 7. Needle holder 4. Conjunctival scissors
Anaesthesia	1. Regional – local infiltration, peribulbar, subtenon
Procedure	1. A single pedicle flap is created from conjunctiva adjacent to a corneal lesion with the base at the insertion of one of the rectus muscles 2. The corneal epithelium is debrided as previously described for Gunderson's flap 3. The flap should be 20–30% larger than the area to be covered 4. The conjunctiva is dissected from the tenons and the pedicle flap placed on the cornea over the site that requires the flap and sutured securely with 10.0 nylon sutures
Complications	1. Operative – haemorrhage, avulsed flap, unable to close the defect 2. Postoperative – infection, ischaemia of flap, persistent perforation
Follow up and postoperative care	Chloramphenicol ×4/day for four days Review at one day, one week, and then as required

Corneal biopsy

Indications	1. Undiagnosed infections with negative smears and cultures 2. Progressive keratitis with an infiltrate that is inaccessible to corneal scraping 3. Undiagnosed but significant corneal pathology, e.g. genetic metabolic storage diseases, degenerations, dystrophies
Setting	1. Slit lamp 2. Operating room
Equipment required	1. Speculum 2. Trephine (dermatological 2–3 mm) 3. Sharp blade (preferably a diamond) 4. Fine forceps
Anaesthesia	1. Topical 2. Regional – local infiltration, peribulbar, subtenon
Procedure	1. Select the site for biopsy which should include a leading edge of the lesion and a portion of uninvolved tissue 2. Outline it with a trephine or blade up to a depth of 0.2–0.3 mm followed by lamellar dissection of the area 3. Place the specimen in a sterile container, moisten with BSS
Managing the specimen	1. Infectious aetiology – divide the tissue into two for (a) histopathology and (b) microbiology 2. Non-infectious – divide the tissue into two for (a) histopathology (buffered isotonic formalin) and (b) electron microscopy (glutaraldehyde)
Complications	1. Operative – iatrogenic corneal perforation 2. Postoperative – secondary infection
Follow up and postoperative care	1. Topical antibiotic and a cycloplegic agent until the epithelium covers the biopsy site 2. Review daily, then regularly until it heals, then as required

Corneal micropuncture

Indications	Recurrent erosion
Setting	Slit lamp
Equipment required	25 gauge needle
Anaesthesia	Topical
Procedure	1. Identify unstable area. 2. Multiple punctures (50–150) with 25 gauge needle
Complications	1. Corneal ulceration 2. Infection
Follow up and postoperative care	Pad/12 hours Seven days, then as required

Corneal scraping

Indications	Infective keratitis
Setting	Slit lamp

Equipment required	1. Alcohol lamp
	2. Kimura spatula
	3. Glass slides
	4. Agar plates – blood agar
	            – chocolate agar
	            – Sabouraud's agar
	5. Liquid media – special brain–heart infusion broth
	                – cooked meat medium

Anaesthesia	1. Topical – non-preserved local anaesthetic preferred – proparacaine hydrochloride (0.5%)
Procedure	1. Remove any adherent mucopurulent material 2. The platinum spatula is used to collect specimens of corneal scrapings at the slit lamp 3. Multiple collections are made from the edge of the ulcer and from the base 4. One scraping is taken for each microbiological medium 5. Allow 20 seconds for the tip of the spatula to cool between flaming and scraping 6. Material is inoculated onto the agar plates and into liquid media 7. Transport the slides and media to the laboratory without delay
Managing the specimen	Material collected is distributed as follows. 1. Gram/Giemsa staining 2. Blood agar – incubated anaerobically at 35°C 3. Chocolate agar – incubated in air 15% CO_2 at 35°C 4. Sabouraud's agar – incubated in air at 28°C 5. Special brain–heart infusion broth – incubated in air 15% CO_2 at 35°C 6. Cooked meat medium – incubated anaerobically at 35°C
Complications	1. Operative – iatrogenic corneal perforation 2. Postoperative – negative results
Follow up and postoperative care	First review no later than 24 hours

Corneal transplantation

Indications	1. Visual – keratoconus, dystrophy, scarring 2. Pain – bullous keratopathy 3. Tectonic – perforation, threatened perforation
Setting	Operating room
Equipment required	1. Corneal graft set 2. Speculum, SR/IR forceps, diamond knife or equivalent, micro tissue holding forceps, tying forceps, needle holder, range of trephines, small bore cannula, 6.0 silk on a spatulated needle (4 crossover retaining sutures), 4.0 silk, 10.0 nylon
Anaesthesia	1. Regional – local infiltration, peribulbar 2. General anaesthesia
Procedure	Superior rectus and inferior rectus suture 1. Posture globe. Eye and microscope to be coaxial 2. Paracentesis, crossover sutures 3. Cut recipient disc with trephine, blade, scissors. Often 7.5 mm 4. Cut donor: punch donor eye on block, 0.25 mm oversize 5. Place donor disc in defect, tie crossover sutures 6. Place cardinal sutures 10.0 nylon at 6, 12, 3, and 9 o'clock 7. Continuous 10.0 nylon or 16 × 10.0 nylon interrupted sutures 8. BSS to a/c to check for leaks
Managing the specimen	Into isotonic buffered formaldehyde
Complications	1. Operative – haemorrhage, damage to iris or lens 2. Postoperative – infection, primary graft failure, astigmatism, allograft rejection, elevated intraocular pressure, cataract
Follow up and postoperative care	1. One day, one week, three weeks, six weeks, 12 weeks, six months, nine months, 12 months, then annually 2. Sutures removed at 12 months

Corneal transplantation in an infant

Indications	Visual: corneal opacity where an optical iridectomy is not likely to be useful
Setting	Operating room
Equipment required	Corneal graft set
Anaesthesia	General anaesthesia
Procedure	1. Superior and inferior rectus suture to posture eye coaxial with microscope. Positioning is sometimes required to expose entire cornea 2. Corneoscleral support ring, crossover sutures, paracentesis 3. Determine optimal size, usually 5–6 mm 4. Cut donor, punch from endothelial surface with 1 mm oversize 5. Excise recipient cornea with trephine, blade, scissors 6. Place donor disc in recipient defect and secure by tying crossovers and placing cardinal sutures at 3, 6, 9, and 12 o'clock 7. Place 16 × 10.0 nylon interrupted sutures 8. Balanced salt to anterior chamber
Managing the specimen	Divide in two. One half into buffered isotonic formaldehyde, one half into glutaraldehyde for histopathology and electron microscopy
Complications	1. Operative – haemorrhage, damage to iris or lens 2. Postoperative – infection, primary graft failure, astigmatism, allograft rejection, elevated intraocular pressure, cataract
Special consideration	It is helpful to administer an appropriate paediatric dose of an osmotic agent (e.g. mannitol) at the beginning of the procedure to reduce vitreous pressure
Follow up and postoperative care	1. One day, one week, three weeks, then as required 2. Suture removal: usually remove half sutures at six weeks, then other half three weeks later

Corneal transplantation with lens extraction and intraocular lens insertion

Indications	Corneal opacity and vision limiting cataract
Setting	Operating room
Equipment required	1. Corneal graft set 2. Speculum, superior rectus suture (6.0 silk), scleral support rings, crossover retention suture (6.0 silk), diamond knife or equivalent, range of trephines, plastic block for punching donor cornea, toothed corneal forceps, tying forceps, needle holder, small bore cannula
Anaesthesia	Regional – local infiltration, peribulbar, subtenon
Procedure	1. Superior rectus suture and inferior rectus suture. Posture globe so that microscope and eye are coaxial 2. Suture on corneoscleral support band, crossover sutures, paracentesis 3. Measure size of graft and cut disc with trephine, blade, and scissors, usually 7.5–8.0 mm 4. Cut donor, punch from endothelial surface 0.5 mm oversize 5. Remove cataract; capsulorhexis with four back cuts (relieving incisions), nuclear repression, cortical aspiration 6. Place IOL (12.5 mm one piece PMMA) in capsular bag 7. Cover IOL with viscoelastic material 8. Suture in graft. Place cardinal sutures at 6, 12, 3, and 9 o'clock. Then either continuous 10.0 nylon or 16 × 10.0 nylon interrupted sutures 9. BSS to o/c
Managing the specimen	Into isotonic buffered formaldehyde
Complications	1. Operative – capsular tear, vitreous loss, haemorrhage 2. Postoperative – infection, primary graft failure, haemorrhage, glaucoma, allograft rejection, astigmatism, anisometropia
Follow up and postoperative care	1. One day, one week, three weeks, six weeks, 12 weeks, six months, nine months, 12 months, then annually 2. Sutures removed at 12 months

Gram stain

Indications	A rapid test for the detection of organisms in: 1. conjunctival smears 2. pus from the lacrimal drainage system 3. pus from glands in the eyelids 4. corneal scrapings 5. scleral scrapings 6. aspirates of aqueous and vitreous humour 7. biopsies of the retina and choroid 8. orbital and periorbital pus
Setting	Laboratory
Equipment required	1. Glass slide 2. Slide/plate warmer 3. Bunsen burner or methanol 4. Sink with staining rack 5. Crystal violet solution 6. Gram's iodine solution 7. Acetone-alcohol 8. Safranin solution 9. Blotting paper 10. Light microscope with $10\times$ objective and $100\times$ oil immersion lens 11. Microscopy oil
Procedure	1. Dry smear on slide/plate warmer 2. Fix by rapidly passing slide through a flame several times. For fluids, fixing in methanol for two minutes is preferred 3. Flood slide with crystal violet for a few seconds 4. Wash off with tap water 5. Flood slide with Gram's iodine for a few seconds 6. Wash off with tap water 7. Decolourise with acetone-alcohol 8. Wash off with tap water 9. Flood slide with safranin for 30 seconds 10. Wash off with tap water 11. Carefully blot dry or (preferred) air dry 12. Scan using low power ($10\times$ objective) and then examine under oil immersion

Lavage of chemical burns

Indications	Chemical injury of the eyes, e.g. alkali, acids, solvents, detergents and irritants
Setting	Procedure room
Equipment required	1. Speculum 2. Normal saline for irrigation connected to an intravenous tubing set or Morgan lens and tubing if available 3. Cotton tip applicator
Anaesthesia	Topical
Procedure	1. Immediate copious irrigation is important 2. Place an eyelid speculum after topical anaesthesia 3. Irrigate the ocular surface – cornea, conjunctiva, and the fornices – with normal saline connected to an intravenous tubing 4. Visible particulate matter must be removed and the eyelid must be double everted to ensure no remaining particulate matter. A cotton tip applicator may aid in removing this 5. Continue irrigation for approximately 30 minutes, then allow five minutes for equilibrium before checking the pH 6. If the pH is not normal continue irrigation for another 15–30 minutes then recheck the pH 7. Once the irrigation is discontinued on neutralisation monitor the pH every 15 minutes for 60 minutes to ensure no residual chemical which will require further irrigation
Complications	Residual solid chemical particles in the fornices
Follow up and postoperative care	Treatment of the acute stage of chemical burns would follow the immediate management

Limbal transplantation

Indications	Limbal stem cell failure
Setting	Operating room
Equipment required	1. Donor eye – whole eye required, preferably with a second eye available 2. Speculum, superior rectus suture (6.0 silk), diamond knife or equivalent, range of trephines, second operating microscope and hand-table for dissecting donor eye. Paufique knife (crescent blade), toothed corneal forceps, tying forceps, needle holder
Anaesthesia	Local or general anaesthesia

Procedure	1. Posture globe – may need superior and inferior rectus stitch
	2. Superficial keratectomy – remove all epithelium and create a smooth stromal surface
	3. Mark inner limits of limbus with 9, 10, or 11 mm trephine
	4. Excise limbus with approximately 2 mm frill of conjunctiva
	5. Prepare limbal graft from whole donor eye
	6. Excise limbus and conjunctiva with precise dimensions of recipient defect
	7. Sew graft into defect:
	  – inlay corneal edge and suture with 10.0 nylon, knots buried
	  – onlay conjunctival edge and close with 8.0 polyglactin

Managing the specimen	Placed in buffered isotonic saline and sent for histopathology
Complications	1. Operative – haemorrhage, unable to precisely match donor cornea to recipient bed, corneal perforation 2. Postoperative – infection, retraction of graft, haemorrhage under graft, failure to epithelialise cornea, allograft rejection, recurrence of original pathology
Follow up and postoperative care	1. 24 hours 2. One week 3. One month 4. Three monthly for 12 months, then as required

Pedicled conjunctival flap to close corneal perforation

Indications	Perforation (or threatened perforation) that cannot be controlled with glue
Contraindication	Insufficient conjunctiva to close defect as mucus in severe cases of mucosal scarring disease
Setting	Operating theatre with operating microscope
Equipment required	1. Speculum 4. Plain forceps 2. Bard Parker no.15 blade/ 5. 10.0 nylon sutures diamond blade 6. Needle holder 3. Conjunctival scissors
Anaesthesia	Local/general anaesthesia

Procedure	1. Topical anaesthesia and subconjunctival lignocaine
	2. Evaluate perforation site – extent, depth
	3. Create bed for graft:
	   – debride all non-viable tissue
	   – maintain deep cornea if possible
	   – develop "vertical" edge to which flap can be sewn
	4. Design flap:
	   – large enough to cover defect
	   – long enough to reach defect without tension
	   – wide base sited on origin of recti
	   – thick enough to provide necessary tensile strength
	5. Fashion flap.
	6. Sew flap into defect – inlay into corneal defect with 10.0 nylon

Complications	1. Operative – haemorrhage, avulsed flap, unable to close defect 2. Postoperative – infection, ischaemic flap, persistent perforation
Follow up and postoperative care	1. 24 hours 2. Weekly for two weeks 3. Then as required

Pterygium excision and conjunctival graft

Indications	1. Visual – induced astigmatism 2. Symptomatic – recurrent inflammation 3. Cosmesis
Contraindication	Minimal symptoms with recurrent pterygium
Setting	1. Outpatient clinic 2. Operating room with operating microscope
Equipment required	1. 6.0 silk sutures 5. Plain forceps 2. Speculum 6. Toothed forceps 3. Diamond blade or equivalent 7. 10.0 nylon suture 4. Conjunctival scissors 8. 8.0 polyglactin 910 suture
Anaesthesia	Regional – local infiltration, peribulbar, subtenon

Procedure	1. 2 × 6.0 silk sutures for traction placed at 6 and 12 o'clock
	2. Dissect pterygium, outline limits of pterygium and split pterygium away from underlying cornea
	3. Excise head of pterygium – preserve as much corneal conjunctiva as possible
	4. Measure epithelial defect over sclera
	5. Conjunctival donor site:
	   – usually upper temporal
	   – measure graft to fit defect
	   – dissect out conjunctival graft
	6. Suture graft into defect:
	   – 10.0 nylon sutures to cornea with knots buried
	   – 8.0 polyglactin to conjunctiva
	7. Check donor site for bleeding

Complications	1. Operative – haemorrhage, corneal perforation 2. Postoperative – infection, retraction of flap, recurrence
Follow up and postoperative care	1. 24 hours 2. One week 3. Three months 4. 12 months

Removal of a calcified band keratopathy

Indications	1. Band keratopathy that is contributing to reduced vision 2. Mechanical irritation caused by the calcified band keratopathy
Setting	Operating room
Equipment required	1. Speculum 2. EDTA 0.05 M (ethylernediamine tetra-acetic acid) 3. Cellulose sponges 4. Bard Parker blade no.15
Anaesthesia	1. Topical 2. Regional – local infiltration, peribulbar, subtenon
Procedure	1. The corneal epithelium is first removed 2. EDTA is then applied repeatedly as a 0.05M solution on a saturated cellulose sponge to the area affected for several minutes 3. The corneal surface is then scraped with a blade or rubbed with a cellulose sponge
Complications	1. Operative – iatrogenic corneal perforation 2. Postoperative – recurrence
Follow up and postoperative care	The eye is examined daily and padded with a topical anti-inflammatory and antibiotic until the epithelium heals

Tarsorrhaphy

Indications	1. Temporary – Bell's palsy, indolent corneal ulcer 2. Permanent – established seventh nerve palsy, chronic corneal and tear film abnormalities
Setting	1. Procedure room 2. Operating room
Equipment required	1. Bard Parker blade no.15 2. Toothed forceps 3. Double armed 4.0 nylon suture 4. Bolsters, made from sterile rubber/plastic tubes
Anaesthesia	1. Regional – local infiltration, peribulbar, subtenon
Procedure	Identify the site for tarsorrhaphy (central/lateral) and the extent required based on clinical examination 1. Temporary tarsorrhaphy – make a shallow incision through the grey line. Excise enough conjunctiva from the lid margin posterior to that to leave a raw surface. Suture the raw surfaces of the two lids together with mattress sutures tied over bolsters on the skin of the upper and lower eyelid 2. Permanent tarsorrhaphy – split the lower lid at the grey line and excise a triangle of anterior lamella. Repeat on a corresponding site for the upper lid. Suture the raw surfaces of the lid margin with a mattress suture and bolster over the skin. Suture the upper lid margin to the lower eyelid edge with interrupted sutures
Complications	1. Operative – haematoma of the eyelid 2. Postoperative – abnormal lid margin giving rise to secondary ocular surface problems
Follow up and postoperative care	1. Temporary tarsorrhaphy – remove the suture after 2–3 weeks 2. Permanent tarsorrhaphy – remove the interrupted sutures after seven days and mattress suture after 3–4 weeks

Tissue adhesive – corneal perforation

Indications	Non-infectious Corneal perforations (<3 mm diameter)
Setting	1. Slit lamp 2. Operating room with operating microscope
Equipment required	1. Speculum 2. Cellulose sponges (surgical spears) 3. Cyanoacrylate glue 4. 27 gauge needle on a tuberculin syringe 5. Gas sterilised circular disc 3–4 mm cut from plastic backing of drapes 6. Bandage contact lens
Anaesthesia	Topical
Procedure	1. Remove the corneal epithelium and all necrotic tissue surrounding the perforation up to 1–2 mm adjacent to the perforation site 2. In the presence of a flat anterior chamber or perforation >2 mm, inject air into the anterior chamber 3. Meticulously dry the site with surgical spears 4. Withdraw 0.1 ml of cyanoacrylate glue into a tuberculin syringe with a 27 gauge needle 5. Dispense a very small drop of glue onto the cornea. Once polymerisation has occurred a bandage contact lens is placed 6. For larger perforations the disc technique of adhesive application can be used 7. Here, a 3 mm plastic disc is maintained on the end of a wooden stick by a small amount of ointment 8. A single drop of glue is dispensed on the disc surface. Dry the site and press the disc and glue into position 9. Cover with a bandage contact lens (usually 14 mm curve)
Complications	Failure to close the defect
Follow up and postoperative care	1. 24 hours 2. Then weekly until healing extrudes glue

15 Therapy of corneal disorders

The general principles of treating corneal disease are set out in the text but only general descriptions are included to avoid congestion with detail and disturbing the relations of one section to another, which is important when aiming to emphasise the diagnostic process.

A tabulated guide to the treatment of specific corneal conditions is therefore set out below. Included in the tables are the common corneal conditions and some others mentioned in passing in the text. The descriptions are necessarily brief. They include an account of the indications for treatment (not all conditions need to be treated and others cannot be treated), a description of the standard therapy and alternative therapy, bearing in mind that there may be a number of acceptable treatments for a particular condition. Common complications of treatment are also described.

- Acanthamoeba keratitis
- Acute recurrent corneal erosion
- Adenoviral keratoconjunctivitis
- Allergic conjunctivitis
- Bacterial keratitis
- Chemical injury to cornea
- Corneal abrasions
- Corneal foreign body
- Episcleritis
- Filamentary keratitis

- Fungal keratitis – filamentous organism
- Fungal keratitis – yeast
- Granuloma of limbus and conjunctiva
- Herpetic dendritic ulceration
- Herpetic geographic ulceration
- Herpetic stromal keratitis
- Herpetic uveitis
- Infectious crystalline keratopathy
- Interstitial keratitis
- Interstitial keratitis (non-herpetic)
- Intraepithelial neoplasia
- Keratoconus
- Limbal dermoid
- Metaherpetic ulceration
- Papillary conjunctivitis due to contact lens wear
- Papillomata of cornea and limbus
- Pellucid marginal degeneration
- Persistent and recurrent corneal erosion
- Pingueculum
- Primary ocular HSV – blepharoconjunctivitis
- Pterygium
- Shield ulcer

- Squamous cell carcinoma of the cornea
- Squamous papilloma
- Superior limbic keratoconjunctivitis
- Terrien's dystrophy
- Thygeson's punctate keratitis
- Vernal keratoconjunctivitis

Acanthamoeba keratitis

Indication for treatment	1. Alter natural history of disease: eradicate infection 2. Symptomatic: decrease pain 3. Decrease disability: reduce blinding sequelae of inflammation
Preferred treatment	1. Antiamoebic therapy: propamidine isothianate 0.1% 2. Cycloplegia
Alternative treatment	Anti-amoebic therapy: polyhexamethylene biguanide 200 mg/ml
Complications of treatment	1. Drug toxicity 2. Hypersensitivity
Follow up	Daily until healed

Acute recurrent corneal erosion

Indication for treatment	1. Symptomatic: relief of severe pain 2. Alter natural history: achieve epithelial closure and prevent recurrence
Preferred treatment	1. Dilate pupil to reduce spasm 2. Pad
Alternative treatment	Bandage contact lens
Complications of treatment	–
Follow up	daily until healed

Adenoviral keratoconjunctivitis

Indication for treatment	Symptomatic: to decrease pain and photophobia if severe
Preferred treatment	1. Prednisolone phosphate 0.5% four times/day then titrate against level of corneal inflammation. 2. Only effective in controlling stromal inflammation. If the stroma is not involved this approach will not help. There is no place for antiviral therapy
Alternative treatment	Withhold ocular medication
Complications of treatment	Ocular hypertension
Follow up	Every two weeks then on topical corticosteroids to monitor intraocular pressure

Allergic conjunctivitis

Indication for treatment	Symptomatic: to reduce inflammation
Preferred treatment	1. Removal of the offending antigen (if known) 2. Topical corticosteroids (short term to relieve acute symptoms). Prednisolone phosphate or 3. Topical mast cell stabiliser – as a prophylactic treatment, e.g. topical lodexamide 0.1% or 4. Topical H_1 receptor antagonist, e.g. levocabastine 0.05%
Alternative treatment	–
Complications of treatment	Long term topical steroids are associated with glaucoma
Follow up	Review regularly if on topical corticosteroids

Bacterial keratitis

Indication for treatment	1. Alter natural history of disease: eradicate infection 2. Symptomatic: decrease pain 3. Decrease disability: reduce blinding sequelae of inflammation
Preferred treatment	1. Antibiotics: cephalothin 50 mg/ml, gentamicin 14 mg/ml. Hourly for first 24 hours, then hourly during the day for three days then four times a day for the next three days. Antibiotic choice modified following Gram stain, culture, clinical course 2. Corticosteroids: prednisolone phosphate 0.5% ×4/day after organism identified and favourable response to antibiotics
Alternative treatment	Ciprofloxacin or ofloxacin as alternative to cephalothin or gentamicin
Complications of treatment	1. Drug allergy 2. Drug toxicity
Follow up	Daily until epithelium healed, then as required

Chemical injury to cornea

Indication for treatment	1. Symptomatic: to overcome pain 2. To improve natural history of disease by encouraging epithelial healing and reducing corneal inflammation and lysis
Preferred treatment	Emergency lavage of conjunctiva Pupil dilation – atropine 1% daily Topical antibiotics if infection threatens Topical corticosteroids (prednisolone phosphate 0.5%) if inflammation with white cell recruitment ensues
Alternative treatment	Acetyl cysteine and ascorbic acid are currently being assessed in clinical trials Amniotic membrane grafting is also being assessed
Complications of treatment	Toxicity. Excessive topical medication impairs wound healing, particularly epithelial healing
Follow up	1. Severe burns should be hospitalised 2. Less severe cases need regular obsessive review, every 48–72 hours until epithelium has healed, then as required

Corneal abrasions

Indication for treatment	1. Symptomatic: pain, photophobia 2. Alter natural history: encourage epithelial healing
Preferred treatment	1. Dilate pupil – homatropine 2% 2. Pad
Alternative treatment	Prophylactic topical antibiotic, e.g. chloramphenicol ×2/day until healed
Complications of treatment	Impeded epithelial healing, recurrent erosion, microbial keratitis
Follow up	Daily until healed One week later and examine angle and posterior segment

Corneal foreign body

Indication for treatment	1. Symptomatic: pain 2. Alter natural history: encourage epithelial healing
Preferred treatment	1. Remove foreign body 2. Prophylactic antibiotic, e.g. chloramphenicol twice daily until epithelium has healed 3. Cycloplegia – homatropine 2% at time of foreign body removal
Complications of treatment	Perforation, microbial keratitis, recurrent erosion
Follow up	Daily until epithelium has healed

Episcleritis

Indication for treatment	To relieve the patient of symptoms of discomfort or redness
Preferred treatment	Topical steroids for 2–3 weeks
Alternative treatment	Mild cases – nothing Severe cases – oral flurbiprofen 100 mg ×3/day or oral indomethacin 25 mg ×3/day
Complications of treatment	Gastritis secondary to non-steroidal anti-inflammatories
Follow up	May have recurrence and is seldom associated with a systemic disorder

Filamentary keratitis

Indication for treatment	To relieve pain
Preferred treatment	Depends on the underlying cause 1. Tear substitutes 2. Mucolytic agents – acetyl cysteine 10% twice daily
Follow up	As symptoms demand

Fungal keratitis – filamentous organism

Indication for treatment	1. Alter natural history of disease: eradicate infection 2. Symptomatic: decrease pain 3. Decrease disability: reduce blinding sequelae of inflammation

Preferred treatment	1. Natamycin 5% drops
	2. Miconazole 1% drops
	   Hourly for the first day
	   Hourly during the day for the second day
	   Then three hourly for the next five days
	   Then as required

Alternative treatment	Other imidazole, e.g. fluconazole, ketaconazole Hourly for first day Hourly during day for second day
Complications of treatment	1. Sensitivity 2. Toxicity
Follow up	Daily until healed

Fungal keratitis – yeast

Indication for treatment	1. Alter natural history of disease: eradicate infection 2. Symptomatic: decrease pain 3. Decrease disability

Preferred treatment	1. Antifungal: flucytosine 1% drops, miconazole 1% drops
	2. Oral flucytosine 100 mg/kg/day
	   Drops hourly for first 24 hours
	   Hourly during the day for the second day
	   Then three hourly for the next five days
	   Then as required

Complications of treatment	1. Sensitivity 2. Toxicity
Follow up	Daily until healed

Granuloma of limbus and conjunctiva

Indication for treatment	Symptomatic: cosmesis, discharge
Preferred treatment	Prednisolone phosphate 0.5% four times/day
Complications of treatment	Elevated intraocular pressure
Follow up	Weekly until lesion has disappeared

Herpetic dendritic ulceration

Indication for treatment	To alter natural history of disease by encouraging epithelial healing
Preferred treatment	Oc Acyclovir five times a day until epithelium healed, then ×3/day for three days
Alternative treatment	1. Other antivirals, e.g. triflurothymidine, idoxuridine 2. Debridement plus antiviral
Complications of treatment	1. Allergy 2. Toxicity
Follow up	Review regularly while on therapy

Herpetic geographic ulceration

Indication for treatment	To alter natural history of disease by encouraging epithelial healing
Preferred treatment	Oc Acyclovir ×5/day until epithelium healed then ×3/day for three days
Alternative treatment	Triflurothymidine ×5/day until healed then ×3/day for three days
Complications of treatment	1. Allergy 2. Toxicity
Follow up	Review regularly while on therapy

Herpetic stromal keratitis

Indication for treatment	1. Symptomatic: to reduce pain 2. Decrease disability: improve vision 3. Alter natural history: reduce scarring
Preferred treatment	Topical corticosteroids with antiviral cover. Commence prednisolone phosphate 0.5% ×4/day and Oc acyclovir ×3. Titrate steroid against inflammatory score. Reduce Oc acyclovir to ×2/day after one week then daily at the end of the second week. Cease antiviral when steroid down to once a day administration
Alternative treatment	Nil
Complications of treatment	1. Corneal ulceration: enhanced viral replication in epithelium 2. Ocular hypertension 3. Allergy 4. Toxicity
Follow up	Initially every week Later every 2–3 weeks

Herpetic uveitis

Indication for treatment	1. Symptomatic: to reduce pain 2. Decrease disability: to improve vision 3. Alter natural history: reduce intraocular inflammation, reduce raised intraocular pressure
Preferred treatment	Topical corticosteroids with antiviral cover. Prednisolone phosphate 0.5% and Oc acyclovir to ×2/day after one week then daily at the end of the second week. Cease antiviral when steroid down to once a day administration
Alternative treatment	Nil available
Complications of treatment	1. Corneal ulceration: enhanced viral replication in epithelium 2. Ocular hypertension 3. Allergy 4. Toxicity
Follow up	Initially weekly reducing to every second or third week

Infectious crystalline keratopathy

Indication for treatment	1. Alter natural history of disease: eradicate infection 2. Decrease disability: reduce blinding sequelae of infection
Preferred treatment	Antibiotics: c ciprafloxicin (3 mg/ml) or G. ofloxacin (3 mg/ml) ×4/day for weeks
Alternative treatment	G.penicillin (5000 U/ml) for nutrient variant streptococci
Complications of treatment	1. Sensitivity 2. Toxicity
Follow up	Frequent observation

Interstitial keratitis

Indication for treatment	To relieve symptoms of reduced vision and prevent further reduction in vision
Preferred treatment	1. Topical corticosteroids 2. Topical cycloplegics 3. Treatment of the underlying aetiology (although often this has no beneficial effect on the course of the interstitial keratitis)
Alternative treatment	Penetrating keratoplasty following treatment of the acute interstitial keratitis has its limitations due to thin cornea, potential for recurrent iritis
Complications of treatment	Prolonged corticosteroid can result in the development of secondary cataract and glaucoma
Follow up	1. Residual corneal haze, scarring, thinning, astigmatism and calcification remain following treatment 2. Prolonged corticosteroids may result in secondary cataract and glaucoma

Interstitial keratitis (non-herpetic)

Indication for treatment	1. Disability: to improve vision 2. Symptomatic: decrease pain and photophobia 3. Alter natural history of disease: to prevent visually damaging sequelae of inflammation
Preferred treatment	1. Anti-inflammatory: prednisolone phosphate 0.5% four times/day initially – after three weeks titrated topical steroids against inflammatory score 2. Antitreponemal therapy: systemic penicillin, if active disease identified
Alternative treatment	May need oral corticosteroids if scleral involvement
Complications of treatment	Elevated intraocular pressure
Follow up	Monthly until intraocular pressure confirmed to be normal on steroids then as required

Intraepithelial neoplasia

Indication for treatment	1. Alter natural history of disease: to avoid invasive neoplasia 2. Disability: to improve vision
Preferred treatment	Topical mitomycin C 0.02% four times/day or 5FU 1% in pulse doses
Alternative treatment	1. Excision 2. Excision and cryotherapy
Complications of treatment	1. Limbal insufficiency 2. Recurrence
Follow up	1. Weekly during treatment 2. Six monthly for the first year 3. Every year after this

Keratoconus

Indication for treatment	Visual disability
Preferred treatment	1. Spectacle correction 2. Contact lens correction 3. Corneal transplantation Contact lenses are required when spectacles are not effective. Corneal transplantation is reserved for those who cannot use contact lenses
Alternative treatment	Thermokeratoplasty in some cases
Complications of treatment	See Complications of Contact Lens Wear and Corneal Transplantation (p. 76)

Limbal dermoid

Indication for treatment	Symptomatic: cosmesis
Preferred treatment	Surgical excision and lamellar corneoscleral graft
Complications of treatment	1. Infection 2. Rejection
Follow up	1. End of week one 2. End of week six 3. End of three months 4. End of six months 5. End of nine months 6. End of 12 months for suture removal

Metaherpetic ulceration

Indication for treatment	1. Symptomatic: to reduce pain 2. Decrease disability: to improve vision 3. Alter natural history: achieve epithelial closure
Preferred treatment	Treat stromal inflammation to improve epithelial healing. Topical corticosteroids with antiviral cover. Commence prednisolone phosphate 0.5% and Oc acyclovir ×3. Titrate steroid against inflammatory score. Reduce Oc acyclovir to ×2/day after one week then to daily at the end of the second week. Cease antiviral when steroid has been reduced to once a day administration
Alternative treatment	Contact lens
Complications of treatment	1. Ocular hypertension 2. Allergy 3. Toxicity, including impaired epithelial healing
Follow up	Weekly until epithelium healed

Papillary conjunctivitis due to contact lens wear

Indication for treatment	1. Symptomatic: decrease discharge and discomfort 2. Decrease disability: maintain vision through continued contact lens wear
Preferred treatment	1. Improve lens care and cleaning 2. Change to new lenses 3. Decrease wearing time 4. Suppress inflammation with prednisolone phosphate 0.1% four times daily
Alternative treatment	Mast cell stabiliser – disodium chromoglycolate four times a day
Complications of treatment	Elevated intraocular pressure
Follow up	Monthly when on steroids until sure that patient is not a steroid responder

Papillomata of cornea and limbus

Indication for treatment	1. Symptomatic: cosmesis, discharge 2. Confirm clinical diagnosis
Preferred treatment	Excisional biopsy
Complications of treatment	1. Haemorrhage 2. Infection 3. Recurrence
Follow up	Weekly until healed

Pellucid marginal degeneration

Indication for treatment	Visual disability
Preferred treatment	1. Spectacles 2. Contact lenses 3. Corneal transplantation Contact lenses are used when spectacle correction is inadequate. Corneal transplantation is used when contact lens correction is inadequate
Alternative treatment	With extreme peripheral thinning an early peripheral lamellar graft may be preferable to a penetrating corneal graft
Complications of treatment	See Complications of Contact Lens Wear and Implications of Corneal Transplantation (pp. 76, 132)

Persistent and recurrent corneal erosion

Indication for treatment	Alter natural history: to prevent recurrences
Preferred treatment	Micropuncture
Alternative treatment	1. Bandage contact lens 2. Therapeutic photokeratectomy
Complications of treatment	1. Recurrent erosion 2. Infection
Follow up	Review as symptoms recur

Pingueculum

Indication for treatment	Symptomatic: cosmesis
Preferred treatment	Excision: leave sclera bare
Complications of treatment	Infection
Follow up	Review until healed

Primary ocular HSV: blepharoconjunctivitis

Indication for treatment	Not indicated

Pterygium

Indication for treatment	1. Symptomatic: cosmesis 2. Reduce disability: improve vision
Preferred treatment	Excision and conjunctival autograft
Alternative treatment	1. Excision and flap repair 2. Excision leaving sclera base 3. Excision and β irradiation
Complications of treatment	1. Infection 2. Recurrence
Follow up	Weekly until healed, then at six and 12 months

Shield ulcer

Indication for treatment	1. To relieve symptoms of vernal keratoconjunctivitis 2. To heal the ulcer 3. Prevent secondary infective keratitis
Preferred treatment	1. Treatment of vernal keratoconjunctivitis 2. Scraping of the base of the ulcer combined with a bandage soft contact lens 3. Treat the giant papillae (as already described)
Alternative treatment	1. Superficial keratectomy or excimer laser may be required in recalcitrant cases
Complications of treatment	Iatrogenic corneal perforation
Follow up	The management is often difficult and prolonged. The shield ulcer may heal with corneal scarring

Squamous cell carcinoma of the cornea

Indication for treatment	1. To confirm clinical diagnosis 2. Alter natural history of malignant disease
Preferred treatment	Excision
Alternative treatment	1. Excision and cryotherapy 2. Topical mitomycin C 0.02% in three weekly cycles two weeks apart
Complications of treatment	1. Operative – inadequate excision, perforation 2. Postoperative – limbal stem cell failure
Follow up	Frequently until healed, then at three months, six months, 12 months and then yearly

Squamous papilloma

Indication for treatment	1. A lesion suspicious of squamous dysplasia 2. Cosmetic (however recurrence is common and tends to be multiple)
Preferred treatment	Excisional biopsy
Complications of treatment	Recurrence which tends to be present with multiple lesion
Follow up	Until healed

Superior limbic keratoconjunctivitis

Indication for treatment	1. To relieve symptoms of discomfort 2. Improve vision
Preferred treatment	Topical corticosteroids. Prednisolone phosphate 0.5% ×4 daily
Alternative treatment	1. Topical application of silver nitrate 0.5–1% to the upper tarsal conjunctiva for one minute then rinse with BSS 2. Conjunctival resection at the superior limbal conjunctiva 3. Thermocautery of the superior bulbar conjunctiva 4. Topical 5% acetyl cysteine in the presence of filamentary keratitis 5. Bandage soft contact lens may be tried in patients unresponsive to other approaches
Complications of treatment	Raised intraocular pressure from steroids
Follow up	Regularly when on steroids, otherwise according to symptoms

Terrien's dystrophy

Indication for treatment	Visual disability
Preferred treatment	Lamellar corneal transplantation
Complications of treatment	See Complications of Corneal Transplantation (p. 132)

Thygeson's punctate keratitis

Indication for treatment	1. Symptomatic: to reduce pain and photophobia 2. Alter natural history of disease: to decrease frequency and severity of recurrences
Preferred treatment	Prednisolone phosphate 0.5% four times/day during attacks – may be able to control symptoms with a lower dose than this
Alternative treatment	Bandage contact lens
Complications of treatment	Ocular hypertension
Follow up	Regularly when on topical corticosteroids to measure intraocular pressure

Vernal keratoconjunctivitis

Indication for treatment	1. Relieve acute symptoms 2. Prevent development of complications, e.g. ulceration and scarring 3. Presence of complications, e.g. shield ulcers
Preferred treatment	1. Topical corticosteroids (short term) – prednisolone acetate 1% 2. Topical mucolytic agents – topical acetyl cysteine 10% – if mucus excess and adherence a problem
Alternative treatment	1. Topical cold compression – temporary relief 2. Bandage soft contact lens – in the presence of corneal involvement 3. Management of shield ulcer is discussed separately
Complications of treatment	Prolonged corticosteroids are associated with secondary cataract and glaucoma
Follow up	Prolonged topical mast cell stabilisation may be required to prevent recurrence until there is a change in season.

Index

Page numbers in **bold** type refer to figures; those in *italic* refer to tables or boxed material. References to procedure summary* include indications, complications and/or follow-up, as appropriate.